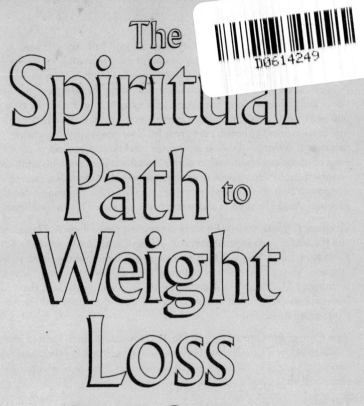

The Spiritual Path to Weight Loss

Praising God by Living a Healthy Life

Gregory L. Jantz, Ph.D.

Publications International, Ltd.

Cover photo: **SuperStock**

Gregory L. Jantz holds a Ph.D. in counseling psychology and health services and is founder and executive director of The Center for Counseling & Health Resources, Inc. A frequent lecturer and guest on radio and television, he is the author of several best-selling books and an audio cassette series. He is a member of The American Association of Christian Counselors, the International Association of Eating Disorder Professionals, and the American Counseling Association.

The Center for Counseling & Health Resources, Inc., located in Washington, is a state-licensed mental health facility that provides services to people of all ages in the areas of eating disorders, nutrition, weight loss, emotional abuse, and a wide variety of other issues.

Editorial Assistance: Robert C. Larson has collaborated with Dr. Jantz on several projects as researcher and co-writer. President of Robert C. Larson Associates, he has contributed to more than 40 books as well as various radio and television programs.

Louis Weber, C.E.O
Publications International, Ltd.
7373 North Cicero Avenue
Lincolnwood, Illinois 60646

Permission is never granted for commercial purposes.

Manufactured in U.S.A.

8 7 6 5 4 3 2 1

ISBN: 0-7853-2786-X

Contents

Preface

It's a fact: Diet fads last about a year. But people who lose weight—and keep it off—know that effective weight management is an inside job and that it's a commitment that needs to last a lifetime. Diets come and go, but those who lose weight successfully no longer allow themselves to get whiplashed by the hype and hoopla of the hucksters of weight loss.

For these and many other reasons, I began to recognize a need for a book like this—especially a book that talked about the *spiritual* pathway to weight loss, asking along the way, What does God have to say about this issue? What is the counsel of Scripture? The more I researched the issue, particularly the spiritual implications of weight loss, the more I realized that losing weight is accomplished from the inside out, not from the outside in. And, in a nutshell, that is what this book is all about: the relationship between body, mind, and soul and the integration of all three that allows us to chart a course for true weight loss and a healthier life, both physically and spiritually. If you feel you have tried virtually every diet imaginable, and each has failed to measure up to its promises, this book is for you.

"Oh," you're saying, "a new, improved diet book?"

No. This is not a diet book. This is a book about you and the weight in your life. I am well aware that the subject of weight management itself may be a tremendous challenge for you, or you would not have bothered to pick up this book. In my more than 15 years as a professional weight-management counselor, I've worked with thousands of people just like you who wage the same difficult wars—often freely described as the battle of the bulge. I hope it's at least a degree of comfort to know that you have not been alone in your struggle. Not only do you have a friend and coach like me to stand at your side to guide and support you each step of the way, but you also have a loving heavenly Father who promises to stick closer to you than a brother.

Your weight-management challenges may seem insurmountable, but they do not need to be. With God's help, you, too, can successfully embark on an exciting, rewarding, spiritual path to weight loss—and when you come to the final page, you will have the head and the heart to stay on this wonderful path for the rest of your life. As your coach and friend, welcome. Together, now, let's embark on the journey.

Gregg Jantz
Edmonds, Washington

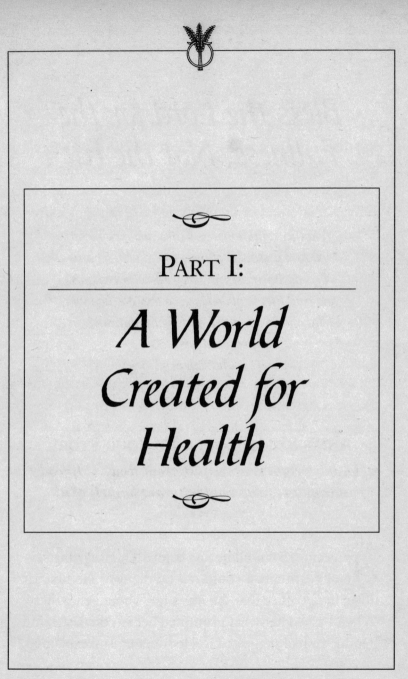

PART I:

A World Created for Health

Bless the Lord for the Fullness, Not the Fat

"And they captured fortress cities and a rich land, and took possession of houses filled with all sorts of goods, hewn cisterns, vineyards, olive orchards, and fruit trees in abundance; so they ate, and were filled and became fat, and delighted themselves in your great goodness."
Nehemiah 9:25

ANN'S STORY COULD BE YOUR STORY

Losing weight is never just about food .... If food meant love, who wouldn't want bushels of it?

Ann came to our clinic just before Thanksgiving several years ago. I could tell by the way she first sat down in my office that she was angry about being there. When I asked her what prompted her to come, she said her doctor had suggested it. Her doctor, Ann explained, wanted her to lose weight before Christmas. "At this time of year," Ann wailed, "he wants me to go on another diet! I'll miss out on all the good things."

I've seen that same look of despair on more faces than I can count when people mention the word *diet*. You yourself may have felt that despair. So I'll say right now: Diets are not the answer to weight loss. That's right, *not* the answer. (Ever wonder why the word *diet* starts with *die?*)

I asked Ann what "the good things" were, and the list rolled off her tongue easily—sugar cookies, turkey dressing, her sister's lemon meringue pie. Then she paused a moment and added, "It's the time of year when we're happiest in our family." Bingo! I knew right then what food meant in Ann's life.

You see, losing weight is never just about food. For Ann, abundant food carried pictures of peace and blessing in her home. It had since she was a child over 50 years ago. Her mother's food, all homemade back then, meant her mother cared about her. For others, food may mean comfort or rebellion or safety. For Ann, food was solid, 24-karat proof of the goodness of love, first from her mother and then from God.

If God fed her, that meant he loved her. The more she ate, the more she felt loved. The more she felt God, or her mother, loved her, the less the other problems in her life mattered—even if her weight caused some of those very problems! It was a vicious cycle. If food meant love, who wouldn't want bushels of it? But the more she ate to comfort herself, the larger she grew. Around and around she went until here she was, at 53, so overweight her doctor was giving her dire warnings about diabetes and heart disease.

Ann is not alone. For generations, Christians have preached that the goodness of God has been seen in the food he provides for his children. What prayer does not include thanks for daily bread? When the children of Israel were wandering in the desert, God came to them in the form of food: God gave them manna. When they grew tired of manna, he gave them quails. The sign of food every day was one very real sign that God was with them.

Since Ann had already indicated she was a believing Christian, I asked her to describe God's physical appearance to me. She looked at me in surprise. I'm sure she didn't expect this question when she came into our clinic. But she thought a bit and then told me. She described a person somewhere between Santa Claus and Colonel Sanders. I knew right then what Ann thought of when she thought of the goodness of God: a short-order chef.

The Journey Begins Here

The journey of a lifetime begins with a single step.

When Ann and I talked about how she felt about food, we began to plan how she would lose weight. This is why I never ask anyone to go on a diet. Both the initial and ultimate false premise of a diet is that *food is the culprit*. Food is not the problem, and, therefore, food is not the cure.

The antidote to dieting—and this is not the last time you'll hear it in this book—is to live a truly authentic, balanced, healthy life as a person who is growing into the individual God created you to be. This is what I want for you. This is what this book is all about. This is the journey you're about to begin. Will it be a challenge for you? Yes. Will there be obstacles in your path? Without a doubt. Can you do it? Absolutely. Of course, you will not be able to do it on your own, and you will not do it overnight. It took Ann several years of steady weight loss to become healthy again. But she didn't start out worrying about those years. Ann began her new life with just one day. Just one day. And then another.

Like Ann, you may not be able to do this alone. Most of us need the strong, yet gentle support and encouragement of others. We all need the help of God. And he wants to help you! Ann told me later she clung to the words the Apostle Paul wrote to the church at Philippi: "I can do all things through him who strengthens me" (Philippians 4:13). She repeated that verse often and put her own version of it on her refrigerator door: "I can get healthy through Christ who gives me strength." I hope you believe that verse with all your heart, because God will give you strength and courage just like He gave them to Ann.

GOD CARES

Sometimes it's hard to believe God cares enough about us to help us lose weight. Isn't He busy with the starving people in Africa? What does He care about me and my weight problems? Shouldn't I just be grateful for all the food He gives me?

Trust me, God cares. Your heavenly Father made you in His own image, and that means you were created beautiful whether or not you see yourself as attractive. When others reject you, God loves you. When you feel bad about yourself because of your outward appearance, God continues to respect you, care about you, and regard you as His child.

LISTENING TO YOUR BODY

Chronic dieters are often out of touch with the biological mechanism that controls their weight.

So what are we really talking about? Is it not the transformation of our inner person? C.S. Lewis once remarked that no clever assortment of bad eggs makes a good omelet. All of the ingredients you need to be the special you—the you God created to be in His image—are all right there inside of you. Sometimes all you need to do is listen to yourself more closely.

People who lose weight permanently learn to pay attention to the body's appetite signals and eat when they're hungry. This was perhaps the most challenging—and most frightening—thing Ann had to learn. Ann became overweight because she ate more than her body was able to use up. Because she often ate when she was not hungry, or didn't eat when she was, she was never able to lose weight. Chronic dieters such as Ann are often out of touch with the biological mechanism that controls their weight. They feel they must starve to lose pounds. Wrong! If you keep yourself hungry long enough, you'll eventually begin bingeing on foods, or your body will start hoarding fat to stave off starvation.

And since there is now a cause-and-effect relationship in place, this pattern will create more hunger as those foods are absorbed, and then still more cravings for the same kinds of foods. The result? A vicious cycle of hunger and bingeing that never stops. It takes the place of normal eating and drives you even further away from what you want most: permanent weight loss.

ANN'S THOUGHTS

If you choose to lose weight permanently, you will also need to review your own thoughts on nutrition and make the choice to become the person God created you to be. Ann told me:

> WHEN I QUIT DIETING, *I began to lose weight. When I started drinking water, I started to lose weight. When I quit drinking three to four diet drinks a day, I started to lose weight. Without anticipating it, my clothes began to feel looser, more comfortable. I began to enjoy my walks around the neighborhood. I also began to eat nutritional supplements—not diet pills—daily that were specially designed for people like me who were in recovery from binge eating. The good news is that during the past two years, I lost over 85 pounds, and I'm proud to say I'm going to keep it off for the rest of my life.*

Dieting and bingeing were tremendous obstacles to Ann's physical health and mental stability. The first step for Ann was to start listening to her body. She had actually forgotten what it was like to eat normally. In the past, she had engaged in so much secret eating, bingeing, squirreling away money for snacks, and hoarding of food that she no longer knew what it was like simply to eat food to provide nourishment and strength for her body. That's why Ann had to learn the art of eating regularly again—three times a day. She now eats a healthy breakfast of light carbohydrates, usually composed of a whole grain cereal with low-fat milk and a banana. It's bulky so it makes Ann feel full. It's also not sugary and full of empty calories. Unlike the old breakfasts of jelly-filled donuts, coffee with lots of rich cream, and other fattening bakery items, Ann's breakfasts now satisfy her until noon, when she can then eat a good lunch without having even to think about bingeing.

But it all started with a commitment to engage in a proven-effective program of permanent weight loss. And you can do it too. If Ann had not chosen to change her views on nutrition, she would have been overweight permanently.

After that first meeting at Thanksgiving when she came to please her doctor, she came back later and said she'd decided—she herself—to lose weight. She was tired of being fat. She wanted to discover the woman God meant her to be. For her, she knew there was no middle ground: healthy and slim or unhealthy and fat. The choice was that simple. She'd already seen what being overweight had done to her health: high blood pressure, the threat of diabetes and heart problems. That same choice Ann made is also yours.

YOU'VE GOT TO GO *THROUGH* IT TO GET *TO* IT

"Therefore I tell you, do not worry about your life,
what you will eat or what you will drink,
or about your body, what you will wear.
Is not life more than food,
and the body more than clothing?"
Matthew 6:25

What Ann didn't tell you is something you need to know. As people who lose weight permanently allow their bodies to go through the necessary physiologic transformations, they also may experience a wide range of emotional transitions. For every ten pounds Ann would lose, she would look in the mirror to see what she was becoming—and liked what she saw. But Ann was not alone in seeing her body's transformation. Her coworkers, including some male coworkers, also started noticing. They gave her positive comments, and paid attention to her as never before. This was uncomfortable for Ann. She was always used to being a wallflower, and she didn't like attention. On more than one occasion she became so uneasy that she reverted to food as her friend and confidant. But with help, and a goal of permanent weight loss always before her, Ann learned to self-correct. She'd come too far in her struggle, had begun to feel too good about herself, and was so confident she was on the right track to permanent weight loss that she chose to deal with all the issues that might otherwise have defeated her.

Ann's weight loss was a journey to self-discovery. One day an innocent comment from a male co-worker really threw her: "Ann, you're looking good...better than ever."

At first, Ann thought it felt good to hear someone say something so nice about her. She loved the positive approval. But it also scared her: "What do I do with this approval? Did I make a mistake in losing all this weight? Have I opened my own Pandora's box?" These were questions Ann never needed to ask before because she used her fat to keep men away from her. We talked at length about her fears, and I reminded her that they were natural concerns in the context of her emotional growth. Ann chose to use the stuff of her daily life to work through her fears, as she continued to engage in emotionally healthy choices; she was discovering that she really could trust the person she was becoming.

In your weight-loss journey, you, too, may find that losing weight forces you to look at issues in your own life. That's because that special you—the person God created in His own image—is an active, alive being. God doesn't want you to step back from living, afraid of being the person He created you to be. God wants you to live your life with gusto, confident in His love and acceptance.

I wish you could have seen the transformation in Ann. As she discovered food freedom, she regained a God-given personal power that also allowed her to grow spiritually. Once pushed back to the outer corners of her life, God now became vibrant and alive. Once socially unaware and purposely inattentive to the needs of others, Ann now searched out those who needed a friend and started developing healthy relationships she never before thought possible. Ann's story says it all, really, because she represents what God can do when you ask Him. She's one of His success stories—emotionally healthy people who just keep growing at all levels of their lives.

Because Ann chose a healthy, whole-person approach to weight loss, she is now able to think about other areas of her life—in some cases for the first time. Earlier, her entire focus had been on food: what to eat, where to eat, and how to avoid dealing with life by eating. Now, food is simply a nutritious fuel to give her the needed strength to become the person a loving God created her to be. She read the verse from the Gospel according to Matthew with new eyes: "Therefore I tell you, do not worry about your life, what you will eat or what you will drink, or about your body, what you will wear. Is not life more than food, and the body more than clothing?" (Matthew 6:25). She realized how much time she had spent thinking about food. But no more.

With her new-found freedom also came a renewed sense of responsibility. It gave her permission to become the boss of her life. No more blame and no more shame. For Ann—and also for you—food freedom means the ability to create and maintain a healthy relationship with all the intricate parts that make her a child of God: the spiritual, physical, emotional, and social person that God created. Ann now has more energy and confidence to do things she had always dreamed of doing but never dared. She had always enjoyed music, but had been afraid to perform in public; she didn't want people watching her. Now, she's taking lessons on the violin and has even performed with the choir at her church. When she packed her diet books in a box, taped it up, and put it in storage, she also put some of her fears away as well. She has now turned to other non-food matters she had left neglected for so long—things her wonderful, caring heart has always wanted to do. She discovered, as you will, that when one works on the development of the whole person, food will assume its natural role.

ONE OF ANN'S ASSIGNMENTS

Your weight is not your cross to bear.

After I'd seen Ann for a few months, I asked her to increase her activity level by another 10 percent, which she did gladly. I also asked her to begin spending 15 minutes a day writing in her journal, where she'd talk on paper about the three deadly emotions of anger, fear, and guilt that she needed to deal with. She would write about anger, for example, under such headings as "ongoing frustrations," "rage," "resentment," and "bitterness." She examined on her own all the different shades of anger that came from her past or were still troubling her in the present. Then, after 15 minutes, she would close her journal, no longer worrying about the grammar or whether she'd dotted all her *i*'s or crossed all her *t*'s. None of that mattered anymore. She was learning that even in her writing, her goal was progress not perfection. She knew she was on her way to wholeness and health the day she looked into a mirror and said, "You know, Ann, I look at you in this mirror today and I really like what I see. You really are becoming the person your loving heavenly Father meant you to be."

As time went by—90 days, six months, two years— Ann just kept jumping off what we called the high dive, dealing with the deep issues of her life such as the hurt, blame, fear, anger, and guilt of the past. It's not been easy, but nothing is easy that's truly worth pursuing. She keeps taking her walks—longer and longer excursions now—and she drinks lots of water. She's become an inveterate label reader, paying close attention to her nutritional plan and limiting those foods that are not healthy. She has become a *dynamic* instead of a *desperate* human being. Just ask any one of her many friends. She has allowed her big, loving heart to come forth and express the unique person she truly is. Ann knows that permanent weight loss is an inside job. The good news is that you can know it too!

Right now, I imagine some of you are thinking, "Great! Good for Ann. But that'd never work for me!"

I wish Ann could talk with you personally and tell you this secret: She thought the same thing several years ago. In fact, she did think it was hopeless when she sat in my office that first Thanksgiving. She thought she was doomed to a second-rate life. She thought she'd never pass a mirror without frowning, never actually look forward to taking a walk. Ann thought her weight was her cross to bear in life. Just something she had to live with. She thought she would always be the caterpillar and never the butterfly.

But Ann—with God's help—took hold of her life. She wanted to be able to walk—just walk—and enjoy it. She wanted, in short, to have more joy in her life. If you have that same longing for freedom, you've already taken the first step in your journey to become the person God made you to be. Celebrate that first step and then keep reading. This book can guide you on *your* journey of discovering the unique person God created you to be.

God Loves You Fat and Thin

*"While he was still speaking, suddenly a bright
cloud overshadowed them, and from the cloud a
voice said, 'This is my Son, the Beloved; with
him I am well pleased.'"*
Matthew 17:5

JENNIFER'S STORY
There are no funny fat jokes.

Jennifer was a classic "fat lady." When she was a child,
other children used to make cruel jokes about her
weight and expect her to laugh along. And Jennifer did
laugh. She didn't know what else to do. When she first
came to me, she didn't expect people to care about her
feelings. Adults were sometimes more polite than the
children but not always. She was used to being
ridiculed. It was either that or being ignored.

I didn't tell Jennifer at first the words I'm going to tell you. I knew she wasn't ready to hear them and believe them. Hopefully, you are. *God loves you. Whether you're fat, skinny, turned inside out, or upside down. It doesn't matter. God loves you.*

I can hear the *but*'s starting in your head already: "But God loves everyone." "It doesn't really count because it's pity more than love." "Sure, God says He loves me, but how can He really?"

Listen close: I'm not saying everything about you is lovable (none of us is perfect). I'm not saying everyone in the world will love you too. What I am saying is that when God looks at you there is such tenderness in His eyes that it would make you weep if you saw it. When He looked down from the bright cloud that day 2,000 years ago and saw His son, Jesus, He felt that kind of love. And that love doesn't end with Jesus; God feels the same kind of love for you today. There is no measuring of love with God. He loves completely and with His whole heart. That's how God loves you. Close your eyes for a moment and imagine God standing you up in front of all of your friends, family, and co-workers and saying, "This is my beloved child, with whom I am well pleased."

"God loves me?" you say. "Me?" Yes, that's what I'm saying. God loves you right now. Before you've thrown out your Twinkies and stocked up on carrot sticks. Before you've walked a mile or climbed a single stair. God loves you just the way you are right now. That's because God sees the *real* you, the you that may be hiding behind a weight problem.

Maybe your problem started years ago; problems of body image and patterning often do. Jennifer's did. She grew up in a family where her parents divorced when she was ten. For years she tried in vain to get the approval of a father whose communication was confusing, unclear, full of unfair fighting, unmet promises, and a thorough manifestation of most behaviors that can stop a child's growth.

Jennifer had no reason to live her life with confidence. Those closest to her—her parents—had let her down, drained her emotionally, kept her self-esteem at a low ebb, and punished her with shame rather than honest, open discipline.

When Jennifer was in her late 20s, she still continued to live out the pain of the deeply ingrained negative messages of the past, choosing not to take the risk of dealing with the emotional abuse that had clouded her early life. When she married at age 31, her life was so out of control that, by her own admission, she wondered if she would survive the first year of marriage. That's when she sought help.

JENNIFER'S OWN WORDS

I don't know how I even made it to age 30. I was so lonely, so afraid, so grossly fat, and completely without hope. But then, someone said there was a place of hope where they helped people like me. So I decided to get help for my weight problem. I was surprised to learn that food and overeating were not my problems at all. I just thought they were.

I had to learn to reprogram my life from its negative past to a more positive, hopeful present and future. But we hardly ever talked about food or my weight. Instead, the counseling was always something like... *Jennifer, have you become a more grateful person? Jennifer, how are you doing in the forgiveness department? Jennifer, you seem to have a deeper respect for yourself and others... Good for you. Jennifer, isn't it great that you can take some time and grieve about your past, but then close the book on it, and open it again to a fresh, new chapter called the present— one you can now share with your new husband, and eventually your children?*

I was looking for help in losing weight. But what I really lost was my unconscious reliance on years of terrible programming that were still making my life a hell on earth. I am now at peace—still a bit heavy—but that is not the issue. It never was. Jennifer has been reborn. I have learned to become my own parent, providing myself with new values that are guiding my life. And if I can make these changes, believe me, *anyone can*—anyone, that is, who's serious about getting his or her life together.

No Shame . . . No Blame

"No slave can serve two masters; for a slave will either hate the one and love the other, or be devoted to one and despise the other."
Luke 16:13

The good news is that you, too, can learn to re-parent yourself, just as Jennifer has done. In fact, you have the best re-parenting tool anyone could ask for. You have another parent who loves you completely, without any of the sins your natural parents have. That parent is God. He can give you the love your parents were unable to give.

God can even show you how to love yourself. The truly mature person becomes his or her own mother and father. Think about the impact of that process: God loves you; He helps you love yourself; and you then become your own parent. This means you get to set the rules. You get to do the self-disciplining. You get to do it all. You can still have respect for your parents or caregivers, but you no longer allow them to be the decision-makers in your life. If you have been programmed for helplessness and hopelessness, now you have the privilege of programming yourself for joy, love, acceptance, kindness, and peace.

The choice is now yours! Addicted to food, you once felt nothing but hopelessness, an emotion we always see as a deep undercurrent in all food addictions. It's a sense of, I've tried and tried and keep failing time after time. You want to throw in the towel of defeat and say enough is enough. Now you are no longer defeated. You have chosen, with God's help, to take charge of your life, making responsible decisions based on your new programming.

It's all your choice. Remember in the Bible where it says that man cannot serve two masters, "for a slave will either hate the one and love the other, or be devoted to the one and despise the other" (Luke 16:13)? You face the same choice. You can't hold on to the grudges of the past and expect to succeed in the future. You can't believe the same old lies about your worthlessness and grow to love yourself tomorrow. You must leave the failures of your past where they belong—in the past.

You also cannot continue to blame others for your problems and still expect to solve the problems yourself. Your parents didn't make you an overeater. Yes, they provided an environment out of which you, perhaps, chose an addiction to food, but they were not responsible for what you decided—and decide—to do as an adult. People who lose weight permanently don't even know how to spell the word blame anymore; they are that far removed from pinning the rap on others. They do not blame their parents, their grandparents, their DNA, their personality, their church, or any other influences from their past. They simply recognize what happened and know that now is the time to get unstuck.

It wasn't easy for Jennifer to give up the lies she'd learned to live with. She'd always thought she was worthless, that something was wrong with her. If she gave up that lie, that meant she was more responsible for the future. She had no more excuses.

THINK REALISTICALLY ... NOT CATASTROPHICALLY

"Far better it is to dare mighty things, to win glorious triumphs, even though checkered by failure, than to take rank with those poor spirits who neither enjoy much nor suffer much, because they live in the gray twilight that knows not victory or defeat."
—*Theodore Roosevelt*

When you are overweight, it's easy to believe that everything you attempt may end in failure. After all, that's how it's been so often for you in the past, so you wonder why the future should be any different. You may tend to exaggerate the negative and assume the consequences of any new action or behavior will be too painful even to try. If such doubts lurk in your mind, now is the hour to begin to turn the tide in your own thinking by doing the following:

- When you find yourself thinking "it's impossible" kinds of thoughts, stop dead in your tracks and ask yourself, Is what I'm feeling based on current fact or old, outdated programming? Do I know this to be true, or am I simply afraid because I don't know the outcome?

- When you find you're afraid of joining the ranks of those who lose weight permanently, acknowledge your fears upfront. Then ask yourself, Am I prepared to be ruled by these fears for the rest of my life, or am I going to take small steps toward personal freedom?

- If you want to lose weight permanently but get hung up on dieting and believing everything you hear and read, go inside yourself for a moment. Ask yourself, Do I have the courage to do what is right for me, even if I do not understand all the details of the path that lies ahead?

The good news is that you already have the courage and the will to lose weight permanently. You don't need to wait for a better time to start your daily 15-minute activity. No time is better than *now* to make your deci-

Reshaping Your Thinking

The following are affirmations that will help you shape your thinking as your new approach to weight loss reshapes your body:

1. God made me an active and alive human being. I am enthusiastically believing this truth as I enjoy my life to its fullest.

2. God made my body to move, not to sit still. That's why I engage in one activity at least 15 minutes a day. I am happy there are no rules for my activity, because this means I can never lose the game. I am determined to be active; I will never rust out.

3. I am excited about my balanced schedule of activity. I do what I can when I can do it. I feel good about myself just knowing that I'm making daily progress.

4. I'm delighted to be active without weighing myself. The scale used to be my judge, jury, and executioner. Now I simply enjoy life.

5. I'm excited that I make no demands of my activity or exercise. I simply do it because it's an important part of maintaining my emotionally healthy, balanced life.

6. I believe the words of the ancient prophet Jeremiah, who said, "For I know the plans I have for you . . . ." They are plans for good and not for evil to give you a future and a hope.

7. I refuse to let external sources get me down or throw me off course. I am increasing my activity level, and my body is responding with a resounding THANK YOU!

8. My attitude is my choice, and I have chosen to lose weight permanently. Nothing can stop me now. I am thrilled that I can enjoy my daily activity for its sheer enjoyment. I feel great!

sion to take action. You don't need better equipment, better weather conditions, better food, better clothes, better friends, better instruction manuals, better affirmations, or better counseling to get better. Just get moving! It's what the people do who succeed in losing weight permanently. They just start moving...and they never quit.

Your new activity will do wonders for your body and for the way you feel about your body. Ninety percent of those who come to me for weight counseling tell me that even the simplest form of activity has helped them feel better about themselves, and that weight loss, which was once their focus, has actually become a byproduct of their renewed sense of self-esteem. What's amazing is that, before long, they find themselves indulging in small, sensual pleasures, such as soaking in scented baths, getting massages, and taking romantic trips—things that never would have happened when they viewed themselves as fat, unlovely, and unlovable.

It's amazing what your new activity will also do for you. People who lose weight permanently no longer spend their time thinking about food, their bodies, exercise, competition, or comparing their progress with others. Their new, liberated mindset gives them—as it will give you—the time to do the really important things in life.

Remember the words of Theodore Roosevelt. I hope you will dare to do those mighty things, regardless of the cost, and despite the joyful pain they may bring at the start, that will be necessary to meet your objectives. Life on earth means there will be change. Growth, however, is optional. The choice is yours alone. God bless you and keep you for your commitment, daring, and never-ending courage as you endeavor to use the tools here to make your success last. It's my prayer that your attitude toward life in general—and your desire for permanent weight loss in particular—may be different for having read this book.

An ancient Hebrew prophet named Jeremiah knew bitterness, discouragement, and despair. His book was even called *Lamentations*. Yet, from Jeremiah's position of grief and sadness he was able to share a wisdom since confirmed by the ages. That same profound understanding of hope for a better future in the midst of pain can also help keep you moving deliberately, confidently, and inexorably toward your worthwhile goals. While this "weeping" prophet wrote of different events, of different people, and in a different time, his words still provide men and women of today with great hope: "Ah Lord God! It is you who made the heavens and the earth by your great power and by your outstretched arm! Nothing is too hard for you" (Jeremiah 32:17).

It is Jeremiah's God that promises to stand by your side and help you bring better health to your body. The more high dives you take and the more willing you are to accept assistance from those who care deeply about you, the faster you will rebuild the self-confidence and self-esteem that God has already given you. There is nothing wrong with you. You are not defective. We just need to change the oil, tune the engine, and put you back in the driver's seat.

You've weathered some great turbulence with diets that haven't worked. You've perhaps exhibited some extreme behavior of which you are not proud. Lightening has struck close by, and you've had some close calls. You may have had your stomach stapled, mouth wired, dieted yourself almost to death, and had everything tucked that could be tucked. But that is all in the past. None of that matters now because you are on an exciting new pilgrimage of courage and hope.

God has preserved you for a reason: to grow into the loving, caring person he designed you to be. Your body has proven to be resilient. This means you can go back and recapture the health and vitality you once enjoyed.

Even Eve Wasn't Perfect

"Therefore do not worry, saying, 'What will we eat?' or 'What will we drink?' or 'What will we wear?'... But strive first for the kingdom of God and his righteousness, and all these things will be given to you as well."
Matthew 6:31, 33

EVE'S STORY—WANTING IT ALL

Discovering how to make peace with our unmet desires may be the single most important lesson to be learned in life.

*B*efore we go a step further, stop and take as your life's motto: *Progress, not perfection.* Forget about your ideal life for a moment, whether that means giving up on losing those ten pounds or ignoring your children's faults. Whatever you feel is imperfect about your life, set it aside for a moment and look at yourself.

What do you see? Hopefully, you see as much of a positive image as you did a negative one—even if it's not perfect. Maybe you've lost five pounds instead of ten. Maybe your children don't call you every week, but they do call you every other week.

Discovering how to make peace with our unmet desires may be the single most important lesson to be learned in life. If Eve had figured that out, think of how different our lives would be! Think about it. There Eve was, living in paradise, and it still wasn't quite enough. The Bible tells us that Eve and Adam were given an invitation to eat the fruit of any tree in the garden—any tree except one, that is. But it was that one tree that enchanted her. Had there been fruit lying on the ground, ripe and ready for eating, Eve probably would not have even noticed. The Bible tells us that when she "saw that the tree was good for food, and that it was a delight to the eyes, and that the tree was to be desired to make one wise, she took of its fruit and ate; and she also gave some to her husband, who was with her, and he ate" (Genesis 3:6).

Why did she do it? Wasn't paradise enough? Apparently not. Like most of us, Eve wanted it all. I can't count the number of times I've read magazine articles about some beauty star who is having plastic surgery because her nose is too big or her smile too crooked. Even truly beautiful men and women sometimes only see their flaws.

Do you do the same thing? Instead of looking at your image in the mirror and congratulating yourself on the shine of your hair, the color in your cheeks, or the sparkle in your smile, your eyes go straight to your thighs or your waistline? We all do this. And no one sees our physical flaws like we do.

Like Eve, we often overlook the good things around us. Instead, we reach for that one thing that we think will make our life perfect. Searching for perfection can be as devastating as dieting, especially because, when it comes to beauty, perfection is not always healthy—and not always beautiful.

I am reminded of an article I read in Newsweek magazine on a questionable "beauty tip" from Japan known as "navel nirvana":

> SUMMER SENDS WOMEN *in search of the perfect*
> *bathing suit, the perfect tan, the perfect...*
> *belly button? In Japan, mid-baring fash-*
> *ions...have inspired some women to turn to*
> *plastic surgery for navel nirvana. For those*
> *willing to hand over $1,000, a 20-minute*
> *procedure can transform a normal round hole*
> *into a "prettier" vertical slit. Tokyo's Jujin*
> *Hospital alone has stitched almost 100 buttons*
> *this year; more requests are rolling in.*

Now, before you pass judgement, remember our own history. In the days when girdles and corsets were prominent, as much as 80 pounds of pressure was applied to a woman's abdomen to make it appear thinner and more beautiful. Today, our teenage daughters and granddaughters are so concerned about how they look that many of them are afflicted with eating disorders.

THE DIET TRAP OF PERFECTION

Diets can keep us from success—from achieving our intended goals.

Reaching for perfection is one of the things that is so destructive about dieting. We tend to judge ourselves as good or bad depending on whether or not we are dieting. Diets create artificial control, and they impose a moral judgment. Diets imply a success or failure. Like the search for perfection, they emphasize what is wrong instead of what is right.

In my practice, I often ask clients to write a journal while they're losing weight. Marsha wrote about a time before she came to see us:

IT WAS FRIDAY NIGHT *and I was going out for a lovely dinner with my friend. I told myself I was going to start my diet the next Monday so I ordered the prime steak with a baked potato covered with sour cream and butter. After all, I was going to be on a diet soon. Then when it came time for dessert, I told myself, "I won't have anything sweet for a long time" so I ordered the cheesecake and convinced my friend to order a piece of banana cream pie she didn't really want. I sat there and ate my cheesecake and then half of my friend's pie. I felt so guilty that I went home and cleaned out the half-gallon of ice cream that was in the fridge. By Monday I was too demoralized to start the diet. I was defeated before I'd begun.*

Diets are among the greatest self-sabotagers of all. Time after time, people come to me with the complaint that they can't seem to diet. And they want me to teach them how to diet, as though dieting is all it takes to achieve perfect health!

Diets aren't the answer. Diets promote competition and comparison. They make us objects—not people—and force us to indulge in self-absorption: "I'm not as thin as so-and-so" comes to mean "I'm not as good as so-and-so." And "I'd better not eat today because I might gain a pound" means "If I gain a pound I won't be as attractive as so-and-so."

When we diet we give our power to others. Our emotions are dictated by what registers on the bathroom scale. Our day can be destroyed in an instant if we wake up, weigh ourselves, and discover we've gained a pound. In fact, one pound is sometimes all it takes to make us upset for a week.

No Extremes

There is no substitute for healthy, balanced eating.

Diets also try to be "magic bullets," deceiving people into thinking that if they can just get the diet right, all their weight problems will be solved. We're in search of that one magic diet that will melt the pounds off. There is no such diet!

To stay healthy, you must understand the importance of avoiding extremes. It takes most people a while to become overweight; it will take some time before that condition changes. Slow down and set some realistic goals. Don't decide to eat nothing but tofu and pineapple juice for a month. Don't buy into body sculpting with liposuction.

Learn to thank God for your body—even if you're overweight and have to puff your way up a flight of stairs. God gave you a magnificent body, and you should thank Him for it. Elaine, one of the women who visits us regularly, has a magnet that she keeps on her refrigerator door that says simply: "Elaine is made in the image of God."

Elaine put that magnet there because she wasn't always thankful:

> I TOLD MYSELF *I was just meant to be heavy. It ran in the family. My mother was heavy. She died at 57 from a heart attack. She wouldn't stop eating her biscuits and gravy even when the doctor warned her that she needed to lose weight. I figured we were just doomed to obesity in my family. The best we could do was hide our weight and go on. I hated my body. Because I hated it, I used it as little as possible. I never walked anywhere. Never climbed stairs. Never enjoyed any physical activity. Didn't even like to be outside because it always involved movement of some sort.*

SEVEN THINGS I DO NOT LIKE ABOUT MY BODY

Complete the following exercise. It's simple. First, write down seven things you do NOT like about your body. Don't think about it too long. Just write down the first things that come into your head.

I don't like my _____ because _____.
I don't like my _____ because _____.
I don't !ike my _____ because _____.
I don't like my _____ because _____.
I don't like my _____ because _____.
I don't like my _____ because _____.
I don't like my _____ because _____.

Now review what you've written. Dwell on the seven parts. Think of them in the extreme. You may have thought your big toe was too crooked, your nose too large, or your eyebrows too bushy. Now you have another assignment. Whatever you wrote above, read it aloud and, after each, say, "So what! Big deal! I was made in the image of God!" Who can argue with that? Not even you can.

If you really look at yourself, the aspects that matter, pretty soon you will forget all about your funny ears or your long nose. The more you focus on individual blemishes on your body, the more you distort your body as a whole. The more you focus on what is not perfect, the more you expand your disdain for your body. In short, you go out of your way to prove yourself imperfect.

Seven Things I Like About My Body

Now, let's try something different. Write down seven things you DO like about your body. Write them down quickly in the blanks provided.

I like my _____ because _____.
I like my _____ because _____.
I like my _____ because _____.
I like my _____ because _____.
I like my _____ because _____.
I like my _____ because _____.
I like my _____ because _____.

How would you compare these two exercises? Was one easier for you to complete than the other? In what way? Now focus only on the seven blanks you've just completed. Read each one slowly and carefully. Look at yourself in a mirror, if possible, as you read each one aloud. You may have said, "I like my ears because I'm a good listener." Or, "I like my fingers because they are long and artistic."

How do you feel about yourself now? When you speak negatively of your body, does it make you feel good? What about when you speak in positive terms? How do you feel when you take the time to be grateful for what God has given you—perfect or not? Do you appreciate what you have?

When Elaine came to me, one of the first things we asked her to do was to complete the "Seven Things" exercises (see pages 42–43). We often ask people to do this because if they hate their bodies, they tend to be self-destructive—eating a poor diet and not getting enough sleep and exercise.

Our bodies truly are wonderfully made, and we are the ones who have reshaped them—not God. When God made us in His image, He did a magnificent job. Imagine a God that can make a nervous system as complex as ours, and still remember to give us little things like fingernails and eyelashes. Take a good long look at your body and think about what it can do. You can talk, walk, eat, drink, love, think, sing, dance, and worship God. That's a lot.

The Bible tells us to give "thanks to God the Father at all times and for everything in the name of our Lord Jesus Christ" (Ephesians 5:20). "All things" includes that nose you don't like and the hips that won't be squeezed into a smaller pants size. It's only when you like your body that you can be good to your body. And when that happens, you'll open yourself up for a whole new adventure: becoming the person God wants you to be.

God Can Use You Now

*"Now the word of the Lord came to Jonah, son of
Amittai, saying, 'Go at once to Nineveh, that great
city, and cry out against it; for their wickedness
has come up before me.' But Jonah set out to flee to
Tarshish from the presence of the Lord."*
Jonah 1:1–3

NOT NOW, LORD

If not now, when? If not you, then who?

You probably remember Jonah best from the Sunday
School stories of him being swallowed alive by the
whale. The main point of the story is that God asked
Jonah to do something and Jonah refused. The Bible
doesn't tell us why Jonah decided not to do what God
wanted. But just think about all the excuses we make in
our day-to-day lives. The excuse I hear most often is
"I'm not ready yet."

GRACE'S STORY

Don't put your life on hold while you try to lose weight.

I still remember the defeated look Grace had on her face when she first met with me. Her younger sister was getting married, and she had asked Grace to sing in her wedding.

> I USED TO SING *all the time, but that was before I gained those 40 pounds. I didn't know what to tell my sister, but I knew I couldn't get up in front of all those people unless I lost 40 pounds.*

When we talked further, I discovered that the extra weight hadn't just put an end to her singing career. Grace also had stopped swimming because she didn't want anyone to see her in a swimming suit. She'd even given up teaching the children's choir at church (something she loved and felt God had called her to do) because she didn't want to appear with the children in front of an audience.

Now, I never advise anyone who is overweight not to lose the extra pounds. Extra weight strains the heart, raises the blood pressure, and can contribute to adult-onset diabetes. But I always emphasize that you should never ever put your life on hold while you try to lose weight.

Over the years we've discovered a connection between weight loss and goals. People with severe weight problems tend to forget what they want out of life. Food has eclipsed their dreams or goals. They no longer feel they have a special purpose in this world. They are in such bondage to food that they've lost all belief in themselves. However, as they begin to lose weight, they learn that their problem is not a food problem. It is a self-image problem, a self-esteem problem, a comparison-with-others problem, a quick-fix problem, or a no-patience problem. To lose weight, you have to slow down, re-evaluate the facts, and slowly change the course of your life.

A LIFE OF JOY

Your body is only one part of your whole self.

If you hate your body, you are likely to damage it—through poor diet, lack of exercise, and low self esteem. This damage is not a part of God's plan for you. God wants you to live a joyous life, secure in the knowledge that He loves you and accepts you. People who live a weight-balanced life don't need to look like the models in the magazines. Your body is only one part of yourself. God made you with a mind and a soul, too. Don't let your body stop you from experiencing all of life, no matter what shape your body is in.

One of the first things to do is to remove the clutter from your life. Find a place that's right for you, far from the maddening array of past guilt, fears, obsessions, and compulsions. In a recent interview, comedienne Rosie O'Donnell confessed that she had ballooned to 210 pounds. She told the reporter that her mother, who had died of cancer when Rosie was ten years old, had become very skinny before she died. Since then Rosie associated being skinny with being sick, and she found it impossible to maintain a proper weight.

Rosie was letting her fears control her life. Intellectually, she knew that being overweight was not healthy, but her fears told her otherwise. Can you relate? Ask yourself how you would feel if you lost a great deal of weight and you looked—and felt—different. If the answer makes you uncomfortable, remind yourself that God is bigger than any of your fears. The Bible tells us, "When the Lord has given you rest from your pain and turmoil and the hard service with which you were made to serve," (Isaiah 14:3) bring your fears to Him.

For others, the stumbling block rests not with fear but with shame. Shame can also lead to an unhealthy relationship to food. For example, even if you're determined to lose weight, if a friend or family member shames you when you slip up, your little indulgence of one cookie may ultimately lead to a gallon of ice cream.

AVOIDING A RELAPSE

"Great works are performed not by strength, but by perseverance."
—*Samuel Johnson*

Someone once said that we humans have a tendency to crucify ourselves between two thieves: the regret of yesterday and the fear of tomorrow. Regret and fear can rob us of precious years of productive labor and love. We cannot change our past, only accept it. It's the regret and the *if only*'s of what's gone before that keep us from living in the present and looking toward the future with excitement and joy.

So how will you stay the course? How will you live a well-balanced life with your weight under your control? Let's look at some proven, creative ways for you to help meet your objectives:

Let discipline start at the center. A man prayed fervently, "Lord, fill me, please fill me." A friend standing nearby said, "Don't bother, Lord, he leaks." When there is little or no discipline at the center of your life, you will leak. A life centered on God is a life that is centered securely. If you wish to lose weight, you will not allow the many distractions of life to throw you off course. Discipline your desires, and be willing to postpone immediate gratification for the sake of a better future. Be optimistic about your progress. Face the mistakes of your past and press on. Be too grand for worry, too hopeful for despair, too kind to hurt another, and too committed to healthy weight loss to give up.

Discipline your priorities. The Bible talks about people who say one thing and do another. Jesus said that just because people say they are in tune with him, it doesn't mean that they are. He told us to look at a person's actions to see what their heart contains. The same applies to weight loss. No matter how good a game you talk, it's only action that counts. Unfortunately, when all is said and done, there is usually more *said* than *done*. Your success depends on how seriously you take your priorities which can lead you to—or take you further away from—your goal of maintaining a healthy weight.

Discipline your nerve. Whenever you choose not to face the reality of life and its many challenges, you weaken your character. General Omar Bradley summed it up when he said, "Bravery is the capacity to perform properly even when scared half to death." Is the whole-person approach to balanced weight loss frightening? It can be. For some, weight-loss success is akin to trying to find a black cat in a darkened yard in the wee hours of a moonless night. You know it's there, but you don't know where or how you'll find it. Don't forsake your dream for lack of courage. Success takes courage, and courage will help you stay the course.

Discipline your follow-through. There are few sports where the follow-through is not vital. This is particularly true in tennis, baseball, and golf. It must all come together at once. It's the only way you'll ever follow through.

There once was a man who sat for days on the seashore, never moving from his spot. Finally, people became concerned and asked him why he never even flinched. He said, "You see, I'm a believer in reincarnation. That means we have lived many lives before, and we'll live many lives after this. So I've just decided to sit this one out." At times, I've heard similar sentiments from Christians who think that being a believer means you step back and let God do everything. They, too, refuse to take action. And it's sad because you will only achieve your objectives and make your dreams a reality if you step up to the plate, take some swings, and follow through; it's the best way to stay the course.

Discipline your time. Have you ever said, "I don't have time"? What you really meant was, "I've not yet made it a priority. It's not important to me. I have other things I'd rather do."

People who lose weight and keep it off know that the process takes time. It's a process that cannot be rushed. They learn what is important is not necessarily urgent, and what is urgent is seldom important. That's why we've mentioned over and over that weight loss is a journey of progress, not perfection.

Ask yourself how disciplined you are about your time? Do you want to be a sunflower, born of the warm, summer ground in a heartbeat, but wilting a few weeks later? Or are you willing to discipline yourself to become an oak tree—sturdy, strong, healthy, and built for the long haul?

While cleaning out his desk one day, a man found a three-year-old shoe repair ticket in the back of a drawer. He realized that's where his favorite pair of shoes had been. He went to the repair shop with the ticket, and to his surprise, the repairman said the shoes were there. "May I have them now?" he asked. The man replied, "I'm sorry, sir, they're not quite ready. Could you come back Friday?"

If you do not discipline your time, it will be a challenge for you to join the ranks of those who maintain a safe, healthy weight. But if you do find discipline, you will stay the course.

Discipline yourself to "what is." This is your reality check. Like a moth attracted to a light, you may be batting your wings at something that will never get you anywhere, as bright and exciting as it may appear: "If I were only younger, or thinner, or smarter, or richer, or had a better background." You will only begin to achieve success when you know how to set your expectations.

In the Old Testament, there is a story of the children of Israel who, while traveling through the desert on their way to the Promised Land, had to live on manna for 40 wandering years. Manna appeared with the morning dew, and the Hebrews were instructed to gather only what was needed for one day because any surplus would breed tiny worms and be spoiled.

Why did they call it manna? Because they didn't know what it was. The word *manna* means "what is." To the weary travelers, manna was reality. And they got a taste of it one day at a time. For you, your manna is what's staring you in the face right now. It's your loves, fears, challenges, joys, and everything in between. When you discipline yourself to what is, you will stay the course.

YOU ARE NOT YOUR WEIGHT

The philosopher José Ortega y Gassett wrote, "Tell me to what you pay attention, and I will tell you who you are." You are not food. You are not a diet. You are a unique person created in the image of a loving God. But as you walk this journey, you will need to remember that you are not what you think you are, but what you think, you are. That's the power of your subconscious mind. Your job is to make it work for you.

Discipline your disciplines. Real freedom is not staged. It flows. It has its own rhythm. We've heard about the importance of not weighing yourself, not dieting to excess, not setting up rigid rules, not buying expensive exercise equipment, not drinking sodas, and the list goes on. All these no-nos may seem rather restricting, but remember, this is a program about freedom, not bondage. In the beginning, you may need to discipline yourself to help your weight-loss program take root. But once these disciplines take hold, staying the course will become a process that seems very natural to you.

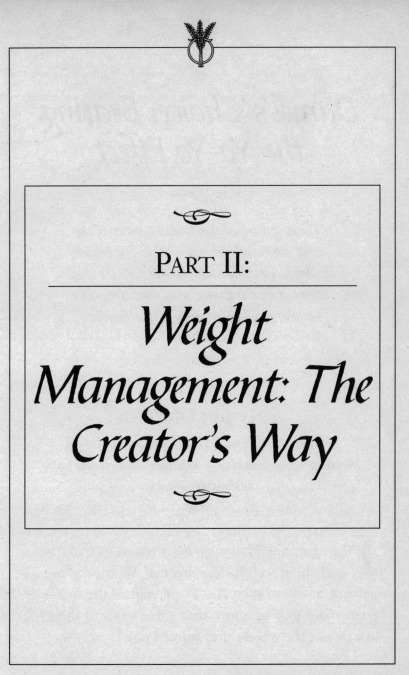

PART II:

Weight Management: The Creator's Way

Daniel's Choice: Beating the Yo-Yo Effect

"The king assigned them a daily portion of the royal rations of food and wine . . . . But Daniel decided he would not defile himself with the royal rations of food and wine; so he asked the palace master to allow him to not defile himself."

Daniel 1:5,8

A NATION OBSESSED

Americans spend $32 billion annually on dieting. An estimated 8 million Americans have eating disorders.

*T*he magazine *Psychology Today* recently conducted a poll about weight-loss dreams. An astonishing 24 percent of the women and 17 percent of the men said they would give up more than three years of their life just to lose the weight they wanted now!

Incredible, you say. I agree. We have become a nation obsessed with weight loss to the extent that a significant number of people would choose weight loss over life itself. What kind of choice is that?

Currently 31 million American women—a number equal to the total population of California—are on diets. And some of these diets are extremely dangerous. It seems that all someone needs to say is, "I lost 20 pounds eating nothing but jelly donuts and wild mushrooms," and there will be plenty of others who will rush out to try it. We have the ten-day diet, the three-day diet, the grapefruit diet, the pasta diet—you name it, and someone has tried it. How did we ever get in such a predicament?

As you have learned by now, this is not a diet book. It's not a book on weight loss with low-fat recipes and not another volume that encourages you to add even more stress to your body through roller-coaster weight management programs that only increase the challenges you already face. Can any reasonable person honestly believe that it's healthy to eat only one food or consume nothing but prepackaged shakes? Instead, the central idea throughout is what we now know to be the only kind of thinking that works: the whole-person approach. An approach that involves your mind, your body, and, equally important, your soul.

DANIEL'S DIET OF FAITH

*Little is much if God is in it. Learn to live a simple
life and eat accordingly.*

~

Do you remember the Old Testament story of Daniel
and his friends? They were young Israelites who were
taken hostage by King Nebuchadnezzar in 605 B.C. The
king provided well for his young hostages, offering
them many delicacies from the royal rations to eat in
hopes of adding them to his court.

Daniel could have taken the king's buffet as his right.
After all, Daniel was a captive; he deserved some reward
for his suffering. For many of the people I see, the
desire to have a reward or comfort for their pain is a
powerful reason to overeat. When all else is wrong in
their life, it is easy to make a donut their best friend.

Not only could Daniel have used his suffering to jus-
tify overeating, he could have also argued that it certainly was easier just to accept what food he was offered.
He could have eaten his fill and not even taken responsibility for it since someone else gave it to him. As it
was, he had to make a special deal with the palace master to get away from the rich royal food. He was, after
all, a hostage. Surely, God would understand if he ate
what was set before him.

I believe we have, as a nation, eaten at the "King's Table" for too many years. I remind people this when they try to offer others "love and friendship" on a plate. We've taken as a national motto that "nothing says loving like something from the oven." But, no matter who you are, *you* are responsible for what goes into your mouth! Don't let your mother decide what you eat; don't let your spouse decide what you eat; don't let anyone else take that decision from you.

Daniel refused to let even the king make that choice for him! It did not matter that Daniel was seated at a perpetual Thanksgiving dinner table with the gravy on his left and the pumpkin pie on his right. He knew that the man who controlled his appetite was the man whom God honored.

Daniel looked beyond food. The Bible says he did not let food *defile* him; but he also did not let food *define* him. He made a wise and thoughtful decision about what he would eat. And, what he would eat, he decided, was what was good for him, body and soul. Since the delicacies in the king's rations had been offered to idols, Daniel knew they were not good for his soul. Therefore, they were not good for his body.

Like Daniel held captive in Babylon, think of your soul before you sit down to eat. Ask yourself, "What is really best for me today? What will keep my body, mind, and soul well today?" Is it really two donuts, or would you do better to eat a plain baked potato and some broiled fish?

That's why we do not isolate weight as a single issue. We don't focus on the use of scales, on exactly how many calories you eat, or on a daily regimen of checking to see how much you've lost or how much you've gained in the last week. The whole-person approach does not encourage you to tally calories or check your body fat, nor are we walking cholesterol or sodium counters. This is because people who lose weight successfully do not rely on the stuff most diets are made of. They are looking at more than the food they eat or don't eat. They are looking at the overall good for their bodies, minds, and souls.

Instead of working toward perfection in weight management, the people who succeed inch toward progress. People who lose weight effectively come to understand that food is not the issue, because if food were the problem, then diets would be the answer. People who lose weight—and keep it off—understand they no longer need to rely on their friendship with food for solace and comfort.

No longer do such people feel trapped and immobilized by weight. Instead they begin to see themselves as individuals for whom the issue of weight is only one component of a complete, balanced life. That is the exhilarating thing about this approach. And that same excitement can be yours.

CAROL'S STORY

Daniel's real triumph wasn't in the fiery furnace. It was gained, first, at the banqueting table. If he hadn't triumphed over his appetites, he never would have had the faith to face the furnace.

While your story will no doubt be different, there may be similarities to the challenges faced by a woman named Carol, a woman I started working with several years ago. Today, Carol describes her life as one she thought she would never live: Her body, mind, and soul are in harmony. She's at peace with herself and her weight.

But not long ago, this frustrated, angry, out-of-control mother realized that if she didn't get help, there would be no hope for her. Food ruled her life. It was the first thing she thought about when she got up in the morning and the last thing she thought about when she went to bed at night. She had a family, but food was her more constant friend.

When I started seeing Carol for weight counseling, she had already been on 13 different diets, none of which had worked. In fact, after each diet fiasco, Carol always gained back the weight she lost, plus a few extra pounds. You can imagine how large she'd become after putting her body through such intense shock over so many years. I'd estimate that since she was in junior high school, Carol had probably shed a total of 300 to 400 pounds and then gained it all back.

She was miserable yet, she continued to begin every diet with a vague sense of hope: "This one will work"; "I know I'll make it this time"; "I'll do it right this time"; "I won't fail again."

But every diet was just another breathtaking roller-coaster ride of self-delusion and false promises, with her depression dipping lower each time as yet one more diet proved painful and ineffective. During and after each unsuccessful diet experience, Carol's highs were high and her lows lower than low.

She had come to the end of the line. Her soul was weary. Her body was out of shape. And her heart was defeated. She now knew that diets didn't work and never would. She'd failed at every diet she'd ever tried, and she began to think that she, herself, was nothing but a failure—a zero. She wondered what would work? Did she have any hope left?

How did this terrible diet mania start? What put Carol on the hopeless path of eating disorders in the first place? What had gone on in her past to create a foundation of pain that dogged her steps well into adulthood? In our first counseling session, Carol told me her mother had started putting her on diets at the age of 13, while she was in the 6th grade. She'd been reduced to eating nothing but celery sticks and carrots with a piece of broiled chicken and fruit for dinner.

At that time, Carol was the largest person in her class. Her peers ridiculed her for her size. On more than one occasion she heard her friends laughing behind her back. She would fight back the tears when she heard them calling her "cow," and "pig," and "monster." Deep inside she was convinced they were right. That was how she looked. Worse yet, it was how she felt about herself. Even though her mother had started the diet, Carol was more than willing to do anything to get the weight off.

Her weight made her look older than she was. She was a child in an oversized adult's body. Since she had no real friends at school, she began to walk down a path I have seen all too often—a journey that embraced an intimate, negative relationship with food.

Carol would sneak snacks during recess, hide food in her desk, and pilfer sandwiches and cookies from the lunch bags of her fellow students. Several times a week on the way home from school, she would pay homage to the corner grocery store where candy, jelly donuts, and half gallons of ice cream were waiting to be her friends. All that food had to go someplace, and without any exercise or care for her body, Carol just got larger and larger.

Her mother assumed the only way for Carol to reduce her weight was to go on a diet, and then another, and then another. After all, the tabloids at the supermarket printed oversized headlines about the overnight diet success of one skinny celebrity after another. The women's magazines she read promised miracles if the overweight person would just eat this, not eat that, take this pill, buy this potion, drink this shake. Whatever was printed about dieting, Carol's mother made sure her daughter tried it, no matter how extreme.

UNATTAINABLE IDEALS

Consider this: The average female model in America is 5 feet, 9 inches tall and weighs 123 pounds. The average woman in America is 5 feet, 4 inches tall and weighs 144 pounds. What does that say about how you feel about your body and where you got those ideas?

When the diets didn't work—and they never did—she began taking Carol to several different doctors in town. They were called weight specialists, but even ritual appearances in the offices of these medicine men and women did not work. So she began buying diet pills for her daughter, thinking surely that pills would do the trick. They would work for a while, and then Carol would get sick, so she'd try another brand of false promises.

During this ordeal she would put Carol on a scale three to four times a day, hoping, searching, praying for those two or three elusive pounds that somehow miraculously might have fallen from Carol's body. But the needle on the scale invariably went right instead of left. Carol would stand on the scale and cry as the scale confirmed what she knew would be true: another one, two, three, four, or five new pounds.

Without knowing it, her mother had set Carol up for failure. She continued to look for the magic pill, the overnight answer, the one diet that would help her daughter shed her unwanted weight, all to no avail. Carol was learning a lot about dieting. She was also learning that her body was not her friend.

People who rely on diets, advertising hype, binges, purges, and pills are living with the same ineffective paradigm. Perhaps this is you. You've been swimming in the same shark-infested waters of weight loss for years, struggling to swim upstream, fighting the tide, and worrying whether or not you were going to keep your weary head above water. Even though you had the best of intentions, you never quite made it. So you took a breather, read some of the latest diet books, bought some expensive exercise equipment promoted by a celebrity on a late-night television infomercial, believed the tabloid headlines, and said to yourself, "Yes, now I've got it. Finally I have the answer." So you jumped back into the water and started struggling against the same current, fighting the familiar, unforgiving tide. But eventually you succumb to the numbing fatigue that discourages, frightens, and sets you up for yet another bout with failure.

It took Carol years to get her weight under control. But it didn't take her that long to see the connection between her body, soul, and mind. She knew that God loved her and saw the struggle she had with each bite of food. She knew she was working to have harmony with her body. Every morning she'd begin her day with a prayer that asked God to help her live a balanced life that day. And she wasn't only praying about the food she ate. A balanced life came to mean a life that focused on more than food, that provided nourishment for her soul and her mind as well.

You, too, can live a balanced life like Carol. I know this may seem hard to believe right now. If you're like most of the people I talk to, you may have already tried more than your share of weight-loss tricks and not succeeded with any of them. That's why I emphasize so strongly that weight loss doesn't come from tricks. There are no shortcuts to successful weight management and good health—physical or spiritual health. The balanced life takes time. And it all begins with one step in the right direction.

Daniel took that step when he rejected the king's rich foods. You, too, can take that step in your life by asking yourself, "What is best for my body, mind, and soul?" Once your heart is ready to make the commitment to do what's best for your body, you're on your way. You'll see what promise awaits in your own life as you live with more balance and learn to throw out the crutches that have kept you immobilized. So turn the page and keep reading, because there's still more good news ahead.

Losing Weight Can't Be That Simple

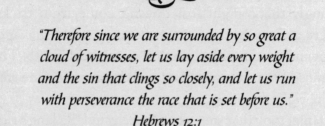

"Therefore since we are surrounded by so great a cloud of witnesses, let us lay aside every weight and the sin that clings so closely, and let us run with perseverance the race that is set before us."

Hebrews 12:1

I Wish...

If wishes were horses, then beggars would ride.

We've all wished for quick-fixes to the problems we face in life, but the truth is, you can't lose weight by simply wishing it so.

However—and this is the good news—weight loss doesn't need to be as difficult as you think. I remind my clients that losing weight is like running a race: The first few strides might be painful and your legs and feet might ache, but once you feel the wind on your face, you'll begin to feel the pleasure of the movement and forget the pain. Suddenly, you'll be running the race because you enjoy it.

It's the same way with losing weight. I see the same process time and time again. Usually, a person starts out feeling skeptical. (After all, almost everyone has tried some type of diet at one time or another and failed.) But after a while, people hit their stride and then weight loss becomes a natural consequence of the new lifestyle they've chosen. That's what happens when losing weight is not the goal—when instead, the goal is to live a healthy life. It is that life that leads to weight loss.

More than once I've even told people to stop trying to lose weight. That's right. I've seen people try so hard to lose weight that they actually pile the pounds on!

OLD RULES DON'T BRING NEW LIFE

You can't put new wine in old wineskins anymore than you can put new life into old rules. Freedom is throwing out the old rules and learning to live with joy in your heart.

Question the old rules. That's one of the first things I ask people to do when they come to see me. We're in the habit of doing things the same way even when they don't work.

How often have you been on a diet that entailed counting calories? How many times have you weighed yourself this year? How many times have you taken diet pills or followed a fad diet? I doubt if any of these diets met your expectations. If it hasn't worked in the past, there is absolutely no reason to believe it will work now! (One definition of insanity is trying the same thing over and over again and expecting a different result!)

Oftentimes the hardest part of being overweight isn't the extra pounds we carry on our bodies, it's the extra pounds we carry in our hearts. People who lose weight, and keep it off, recognize the pain in their hearts.

Remember Carol from the previous chapter? She realized there were many unkind people in her life who had judged her unfairly—starting with her classmates in junior high school. Later it was uncaring neighbors, relatives, and acquaintances. These critics believed that because Carol was overweight there must be something wrong with her. Carol no longer believes that, but at one point she did, and the heaviness of that belief—and the resentment towards those who criticized her— weighed more on her than the extra pounds she carried.

I remember her first days with me. Shortly after we began talking together I asked her to record her

FREEDOM FROM THE RULES OF DIETING

One of the challenges St. Paul faced was similar to one we deal with when we try to lose weight: to change our old ways of thinking. The religious people in Paul's day believed that if you wanted to get into heaven, you had to follow certain rules—the Mosaic Law. Then Jesus came along and changed all the rules. In his letter to the Romans, St. Paul wrote:

> WHILE WE WERE *living in the flesh, our sinful passions, aroused by the law, were at work in our members to bear fruit for death. But now we are discharged from the law, dead to that which held us captive, so that we are slaves not under the old written code but in the new life of the spirit. (Romans 7:5–6)*

Imagine the confusion. Now it didn't matter how many steps you had taken because that road no longer led to heaven. People had to learn to accept a new way of looking at things. They needed to throw out all the old rules and start anew. Not only did Paul say that the rules were a hindrance; he actually lays the blame at their feet—the rules are the problem itself. People who lose weight effectively learn that weight loss comes through personal freedom and a lack of rules. Rules kill; freedom gives birth to personal growth. Rules immobilize; freedom gives you hope to last a lifetime. This same kind of freedom allows you to lose weight.

thoughts of those early days, and she has agreed to share them with you:

DR. JANTZ SAID *he'd like me to conduct a 30-day experiment. I said I was open to almost anything at this point, but what he suggested seemed so bizarre that I almost laughed. First, he asked me to bring my scale to our next session. My scale? My trusty security blanket? A thousand times no, I said to myself. But a week later, I brought it in, feeling very foolish as I muscled it into the office in a large, plain, brown paper bag, as if I were a kind of felon waiting to be caught for smuggling contraband. I was told my scale had simply gone on vacation, and that I could have it back any time I wanted it. I thought this was fairly strange therapy, but I promised to go along with it. Then, Dr. Jantz asked me to make an agreement with him that I would do three things on a regular basis. Here is what he asked me to do:*

FIRST . . . I WAS TO START EATING *a simple, healthy breakfast each morning. That was my only guideline: It had to be healthy. No list of special foods, no restrictive diet, no number of* calories to count, lie about, or eat—nothing. What surprised me was that I was told to make my own decision and not rely on someone else's idea of what I should eat. I was given complete freedom to eat when I wanted and how much I wanted. It just had to be healthy.

THE SECOND THING I was asked to do was even more amazing. I was not to weigh myself at all in between sessions. I'd already sent my scale "on vacation," so there was no way to weigh myself at home. But I was not to weigh myself anywhere: not at the home of a friend, not on a public scale, not downtown where they sell scales—nowhere. This was difficult. How was I to know if I was making any progress if I couldn't weigh myself two or three times a day as I'd done most of my life? I didn't understand it, but I said I'd be a good person and obey the rules.

THE THIRD THING I said I'd do was something I had not done in years. Exercise. After I had received a complete medical evaluation, everything was set to go. But still, when you're over 200 pounds and gaining fast, the last thing on earth you want to do is exercise. Lifting a finger to help a friend was too much work for me.

*I certainly wasn't going to be seen in a health
club with those trim, young things doing aerobics as if they were made out of willows. But
Dr. Jantz told me my activity would require
no money, no club membership fees, no time,
no expensive equipment, and no detailed book
of instructions. Here was my assignment:
Engage in an enjoyable activity each day.
Choose whatever you want, and do it for as
long as you like, but it has to move your body,
and it has to be fun for you. What was this
weight-loss professional talking about? I asked
myself. How was I going to lose weight permanently unless it was (1) hard work, (2) no fun,
(3) expensive, and (4) something that would
take all my time and embarrass me in the
process?*

In our counseling sessions, Carol and I never focused
on her weight. In fact, we seldom talked about it. We
did, however, address the emotional poisons she had
chosen to live with for so long and offered her a way of
healthy escape. Carol—just like the early Christians of
Paul's day—finally discovered the freedom of throwing
out the old rules and learned to live with joy and freedom in her heart. When Paul talked to the early Chris-

tians about living a new life with a new hope in God, he couldn't have seen a more radical change than the one I saw in Carol. She hardly even noticed she was losing weight because she was so relieved to unload some of the hurt and resentment she had carried around inside her for years. Now, just as Carol did, I urge you to look inside your own life and past experiences.

TAKING A LOOK INSIDE

Food is not the cure for your pain.

What emotional toxins are you living with? What pain, fear, or frustration has become a part of your inner self? If you have chosen food as your weapon against these toxins you are probably aware that you are losing the weight-loss battle. You will only struggle on in vain.

You need to realize that food is not a cure for your pain. And the tangle, deceit, and empty promises of diets will only further confuse and exacerbate the challenges you face. The key to a better, more hopeful future is to deal with your pain and address your real problems if you desire to lose weight and keep it off.

"But Dr. Jantz," you say, "you don't know my mother, or father, or brother, or aunt. It's not easy being around them. They're always judging me because of my weight, telling me about the latest diet and making me feel bad about myself."

No, I don't know your relatives, but on the other hand, maybe I do—I hear about them every day. For example, Carol's mother, now in her 80s, remains obsessed with food and dieting. She has become a master of knowing how to take that prickly thorn of judgment and wiggle it deep into her daughter's side: *You're still not good enough, Carol. Come on, here's another diet for you. You're starting to gain again, little one. Isn't it time we see another doctor about your weight?*

Though this is still hard for Carol to hear, she's continued to keep her commitment to forgiving her mother. Her mother's abusive comments sting but no longer destroy her because Carol has dealt with the real issues in her life. Participating in the false promises of her mother and the deceit of a $30-billion weight-loss industry are no longer of importance to her.

Carol has learned that a lean body is not the answer to the stresses of life. She knows who she is and what place she has in God's heart. And no longer does Carol pay inordinate attention to every morsel of food she eats. She does not even exercise compulsively.

She has learned that the weight and shape of her body are not the determining factors of who she is and what

Out with the Old

Beginning now, you can choose to refuse to be a victim of diet programs. The following action plan will help you get started.

1. You no longer need to weigh yourself because your weight is no longer the issue. Ask yourself: Do I want to weigh a certain amount, or do I want to feel good about myself and my life? Here's what to do: Put your bathroom scale in a closet or in the attic. Avoid using it. It's a crutch—you don't really need it to lose weight.

2. If you have unopened, pre-packaged diet food that's been in your cupboard for months or perhaps even years, wrap it up and put it in the box. You don't need this food anymore. Diet food is also a crutch—you don't need pre-packaged foods to lose weight.

3. You may have items of clothing you've been hanging onto. It may be a pair of jeans or shorts you wore in high school, or a bathing suit that made you look terrific when you were 21. Put all those items of clothing in a box along with the pre-packaged food. Secure the box with sturdy strapping tape.

4. Now, place the sealed box in your attic or storeroom where you know you can get to it if necessary. Then, in big black letters, write on the box, "FALSE CRUTCHES." Put today's date on the box. Remind yourself you no longer need those external tangibles to help you lose weight. However, if you ever feel you need to wear or eat what's in the box, go get it and open it up. We're not taking anything away from you. We are only creating distance between you and the clutter that is guaranteed to impede your progress.

she is becoming. This is what every person who loses weight permanently learns. This is also what every person learns when they accept themselves and learn to rely on God rather than the critical eye of others.

THROW YOUR CRUTCHES ASIDE

Food isn't always to blame.

Diets taught Carol—and teach us all—to regard food as the source of our weight problems. But food isn't always the issue. It is the dieting that chips away at our self-esteem: Diets take the dieter on a roller-coaster ride of false hope and empty promises. Diets have a tendency to eat away at the best of who you are—without you even knowing it.

The good news is that there is hope that you can—and will—succeed in losing weight forever. You now know that losing weight is really an inside job that begins with hope for a better, more balanced life.

People who lose weight effectively take the initiative to begin living from the inside out. Remember when Jesus asked the lame man if he'd like to be healed? You, too, can throw your crutches away and begin living a healthy, balanced life.

When Letting Yourself Down Feels Like Your Biggest Exercise

"Beloved, I do not consider that I have made it my own; but this one thing I do: forgetting what lies behind and straining forward to what lies ahead, I press on toward the goal for the prize of the heavenly call of God in Christ Jesus."

Philippians 3:13–14

"I can do all things through him who strengthens me."

Philippians 4:13

These two verses, written by the Apostle Paul, are among my favorites. They contain some important secrets for us as we walk the spiritual path to better eating and weight management. First, when you decide to lose weight, you must leave the past behind and look to the future. Your past failures with exercise and weight control are absolutely irrelevant. Why? Because you can do all things—now, today—through Jesus Christ who strengthens you. *All things* includes living a balanced, healthy life that is not controlled by excesses. *All things* includes living a life filled with joyful movement and breathing-hard exercise.

Now, I want you to read St. Paul's words three times as you think about your weight-loss hopes. And then be quiet for a moment. If you're like most people, it'll only take a second or two for the *but*'s to show up:

But I already tried. But I can't today. But it never works.

The list goes on. That's why Paul didn't just say we can do all things through Christ. He first told people that it is possible to start anew. Starting anew means for-

COMFORT AND STRUCTURE

Acts 9:31 talks about "living in the fear of the Lord and in the comfort of the Holy Spirit." I am more and more convinced that knowing those two powers is the only way to have a healthy, balanced life in all areas—not just the physical realm. We all need comfort and structure in our lives. If we are lacking either, we are lopsided; when we have both, we are well on the road to healthy, God-centered living.

getting about the old *but*'s of yesterday. This chapter is about letting go of those old obstacles and restoring your own God-given personal power.

Never again do you need to be controlled by external forces to lose weight. You don't need to be controlled by anything other than the Holy Spirit who has been assigned to you as a comforter and friend for all the areas of your life—including your weight.

JOHN'S STORY

*Habit is either the worst of masters or
the best of servants.*

᠊ᡃᡃᢣᢇᠵ᠊

I've discovered it isn't always easy at first glance to tell who is really serious about losing weight. Sometimes it appears that someone is peddling as hard as he can when, in fact, he is just marking time. John is a good example.

When I met John, he told me, with some pride, that he'd just joined his fourth health club. (I thought perhaps he was doing a survey of the various gyms in town.) John was very particular about which health club he would attend. He told me he was determined to lose the extra 100 pounds he carried around, and he was sure the right health club would be just the thing he needed to do that. I wished John well but told him to come see me if he decided his health club didn't live up to his expectations.

I suspected John was doing something I've seen many times—chasing one good idea after another until the idea is the goal instead of weight loss. I've seen that pattern so often in others. I later found out I was right.

John was so excited about the enormous possibilities his new fitness center had to offer. This fat-burning factory was complete with floor-to-ceiling mirrors, the latest design of stair climbers, a simulated rock wall, treadmills, bicycles, racquetball, squash, free weights, and what seemed like an acre of exercise machines promising miracles for people with weight problems. The club also boasted a huge aerobics room where John told me the pounds would probably start dropping off the moment he completed his first session. According to John, the club also had the best, most expensive personal trainers in the area, a juice bar second to none, and a state-of-the-art fitness program that had been proven effective in other areas of the city.

On and on he went. He was so enthused about his new-found opportunity to get fit that I thought he must have been one of the investors. He bought some of my books and a few audio tapes and said he knew all this would help him as he continued on his way to a life of thinness. In fact, he was going to start listening to my tapes on the stationary bicycle first thing Monday. I never saw John again. But I did hear about him through a friend. Here's the rest of the story:

FOUR HEALTH CLUBS = TOO MANY!

The way to get anywhere is to start from where you are.

❧

I learned that John not only had joined his fourth health club, but that he still belonged to the other three. Never mind that he didn't use them. They were too old and needed painting, the equipment wasn't up-to-date enough, there were no juice bars, the trainers were just OK, and besides, parking wasn't all that great; John had to walk too far from his car to get to the gym. For John, exercise only began when he gave the desk clerk his card, suited up, and got on the machines. No one was more pleased than John when the new fitness center came to town. Perhaps this one will do the trick, he thought. I'm not losing weight any place else, so it must be those other clubs. It can't be my fault. Finally, I've found a gym that will work for me.

I learned that John had been on nine different diets during the previous two years. His hobby seemed to be looking for and eating the latest in specially prepared, expensive packaged diet foods, hoping the next name brand would finally provide the secret to significant weight loss.

Good old John was also a regular at the weekly overeaters support group. Whenever he saw a television campaign for a new diet or diet product, he was among the first to line up at the health food store to try it. While he was there, he always picked up a few new books on dieting, stretching, weight lifting, vitamins, and minerals.

But the story doesn't stop there.

It's now Friday. John has become a charter member of the new club. He's received his temporary card, has taken the grand tour, and has even met the owners. He feels part of the establishment. He's been accepted. John says he especially likes all the lotions and potions in the men's locker room. ("Hey, even if I don't lose a lot of weight, I'm sure going to smell good.") John made an appointment to start his new fitness program the following Monday.

Unfortunately, there's something between Friday and Monday called a weekend, and John loves weekends. But this one would be special, a sort of celebration for what he knew would happen on Monday at the crack of dawn with his new trainer. So what do you do when you celebrate? Eat. In fact, you eat a lot. ("If I'm going to have a last meal before the big program, it's going to be a big one.") So John binges all weekend, and really eats big on Saturday night. In fact, he eats as if there's no tomorrow. ("Hey, I owe myself this food, especially if I'm going to deprive myself of what I want to eat in the weeks ahead.")

By Monday, John felt so bloated he postponed his meeting with his trainer. He wanted to be in better shape for his first session.

So what's the answer? John was so caught up in perfecting what he thought he ought to do—he ought to exercise, and he ought to do it in the perfect setting— that he completely forgot the first thing to know about exercise: Exercise should be fun. Exercise does not need to be expensive. It does not need to be trendy. It does not need to involve lots of decision-making or shopping around for specific equipment or juice bars. It's really very simple: The only thing you need is you and awareness of your body.

The questions people who lose weight effectively ask themselves are, What does my body need today? What kind of food shall I eat? What sort of exercise is most appropriate? What kind of activity level is best for me?

Not, what am I supposed to do because I saw 30 minutes of hype on a late-night infomercial or read about the latest, greatest overnight diet sensation in a popular magazine. And when it comes specifically to exercise, the most important questions people who lose weight ask are, How can I make exercise fun again? What can I do that is so enjoyable that I'll look forward to doing it day after day, week after week, year after year?

The way to get anywhere is to start from where you are. Don't wait to exercise until you have the ultimate set-up or have the right clothes, the right equipment, or the perfect weather. There's no day more perfect than today to exercise.

Exercise must be something fully compatible with you and your personality. If you hate to run, don't run. (If you hate it, you won't do it, and so, why should you?) If a sweaty, inconvenient five-day-a-week regimen in a local fitness club is not for you and your schedule, don't do it.

That was John's problem. He'd conned himself into believing that he had to go for a big weight-loss program in a big club, with big fees, big trainers, and big, expensive equipment, or do nothing at all. Unfortunately, John chose nothing, and therefore he may never learn to live a balanced, healthy life.

No More Guilt, Thank You

There are no rules for exercise. Absolutely none!

Exercise is not about feeling guilty for what you can't, or choose not to, do. The guiltier you feel, the less exercise you will do; the less exercise you do, the guiltier you will feel; and your guilt cycle will produce depression, confusion, and anger to the point where your entire system may simply close down. The solution: Do what is right for you.

Choose an activity that is fun. For many people, the best initial exercise program is simply to walk more. Walking requires no expensive club dues, no unique clothing, no time limits, no stop watches, no subscriptions to fitness magazines, no nothing. With walking there are also no excuses. If it's hot, walk early. If it's raining, wear a raincoat or carry an umbrella; then come home and take a hot shower. It's one of the most invigorating feelings ever. Some people find a walking buddy and find that they really look forward to time with their friend. Others listen to music while they walk. The key is to find something you like and do it.

People who lose weight permanently know this. They exercise appropriately, but they do exercise. Some join health clubs and go through unbelievable routines—but they do it according to their own rules. Others just walk a few minutes a day, ride a stationery bike a few minutes a day, lift some light weights a few minutes a day—but when it fits into their own schedule.

A mounting pile of evidence tells us that walking is a good path to healthy living. Remember, there are no hard and fast rules. Any walking you do is better than no walking. If you used to drive three blocks to the store and now you walk, good for you! If you used to take the elevator at work and now you take the stairs, good for you! Every activity you do counts toward your total health.

One day in the future you may want to maximize your walking by playing with the idea of walking three or four miles an hour on a regular basis. Your body will thank you, and over the long haul, you will discover increasingly improved health. But it's not a rule that you do this. Only do it if you want to. Yes, there is scientific evidence that proclaims you must drive your heart rate to at least 60 percent of its maximum for 20 minutes to an hour by running, cycling, or swimming to be in the low-vigorous range. But this may not be for you now—or ever. People who lose weight effectively know that weight loss is all about personal freedom and liberation, never a set of rules set down by others.

People who learn to live a healthy, balanced life say goodbye to extreme behavior in every area of their lives—including what they do for their daily activity. Most people who start out vowing they're going to run four miles a day when they used to drive everywhere, don't last more than a few days. Set goals you'll look forward to completing. Then be patient with yourself. People who lose weight make small, daily steps toward their goals because they know that inch-by-inch virtually anything is possible. Once you decide what your activity level will be, I encourage you simply to increase it a little each month. You'll be amazed at your progress within only a few months.

The main thing to remember—and this is not just true of exercise but of the foods you eat as well—is that there is no magic bullet. There is no machine that will do the work of exercise for you. There is no health club that will automatically make you maintain a healthy life just by buying a membership. Remember the children's story about the hare and the tortoise. The tortoise won the race because he kept taking small steps toward the goal line and the hare raced around until he grew tired and never finished. In weight loss, the tortoises win.

Don't make a big plan. Make a small plan that you will stick to, and then add to the small plan when you've made it a habit. Remember, you are walking a spiritual path, and any path is to be taken one step at a time.

I Know You Hate Celery, But...

"Now John was clothed with camel's hair, with a leather belt around his waist, and he ate locusts and wild honey."

Mark 1:6

WHAT'S FOR DINNER?

John the Baptist ate to live; he did not live to eat.

You've read about John the Baptist, and you've probably shaken your head in disbelief. You just can't imagine someone having a steady diet of grasshoppers—even if he did use a little honey to help get them to go down! Most of us plan our menus more carefully than that! I know I do.

But apparently, John didn't plan his menus at all. He just ate what he grabbed along the way. He would have eaten Big Mac's as readily as those grasshoppers if there had been golden arches around him instead of insects. If he could catch it, he'd eat it. John just couldn't be bothered with his food. He had other things on his mind. He knew God would provide for him and that was all he needed to know.

Fortunately, God provides us with many exciting food choices each day—and, at least for most Americans, insects are not among them. Unfortunately, God has placed more food within our grasp than is healthy for us to eat. As the bumper sticker reads: So many morsels; so little time.

While I am not advocating that anyone adopt the "if you see it, eat it" style of John the Baptist, I do suggest that we might learn some things from his attitude toward food. The main lesson we can learn from his diet is that food was not the focus of John's life, and it need not be the focus of yours either. John was eating grasshoppers because he could not be bothered with taking time to plant grain, harvest grain, mill grain, and then make bread.

John ate to live; he did not live to eat. John was busy serving his master; and his master was not his own hunger. Food was his servant, not his friend or his mother or his lover.

A NEW RELATIONSHIP

"When Jesus saw him lying there and knew he had been there for a long time, he said to him, 'Do you want to be made well?'"
John 5:6

~

You've already heard me say it, but I want to say it at least one more time: Losing weight is not about dieting because weight problems are often not about food. When you are serious about losing weight, you will demand of yourself that you develop a new relationship with food—which may actually mean taking a fresh, new look at life in general. That's because the energy you spend focusing on food, on eating, and on dieting is energy that may be taking away from other areas of your life.

When people with eating disorders come to see me, I ask them how much time they think about food. Many say, "Oh, about 110 percent of the time." That's the most honest statement they'll ever make during treatment. They do spend the majority of the time thinking about food—*when* they are or are not going to eat, *what* they are or aren't going to eat, and *where* they are or are not going to eat. But the feeling of control these individuals think they have is nothing but an illusion. In fact, the eating disorder is controlling them, consuming their relationships, ruining their self-esteem, destroying their health, and wasting their time.

This is what we can learn from John the Baptist: Food is sustenance. We need food to live. Praise God, for He provides us with that food. But throughout the Bible the message about food is this—do not put your faith in food. Food will not love you. Food will not heal your pain. Food will not help you manage your anger.

It's time to put food in it's place in your life.

This is when many of my friends with serious weight challenges get nervous. They'll shout "Amen!" to the compelling ideas and the motivational stories of the success of others. But when it comes time to talk about their own attitude toward food—and what they do or don't do—they start getting nervous.

But please relax. I am not asking you to make a rigid set of rules. I'm not telling you to eat nothing but celery sticks or that you can never enjoy a cupcake again. You've probably already tried extreme diets like that and failed. That's what diets demand: an all-or-nothing extreme kind of thinking—and we know diets don't work. Diets create a system of fear, guilt, and deprivation. Diets are a roller-coaster ride of exuberant determination followed by the depths of failure and guilt. That's no way to eat—or live! No, what we're talking about is how to help you deal with your low impulse control and how you use food as a weapon in a battle you simply cannot win. An overweight person's relationship with food needs to be an art, and it can be learned.

How is it an art? When you choose to believe that you do not need any artificial structures—such as diets—in your life to lose weight effectively, you are ready to begin. Thinking thin doesn't work because it's not a thinking problem. It's a whole-person problem. People who lose weight understand they need a paradigm shift of the highest order. A *paradigm shift* is when you look at some familiar thing completely differently. One of my favorite stories illustrates what a paradigm shift is:

Two battleships assigned to the training squadron had been at sea on maneuvers in heavy weather for several days. The visibility was poor with patchy fog, so the captain remained on the bridge keeping an eye on all activities.

Shortly after dark, the lookout on the wing of the bridge reported, "Light, bearing on the starboard bow."

"Is it steady or moving astern?" the captain called out.

The lookout replied, "Steady, captain," which meant they were on a dangerous collision course with that ship.

The captain then called to the signalman, "Signal that ship: We are on a collision course; advise you change course 20 degrees."

Back came a signal, "Advise that *you* change course 20 degrees."

The captain said, "Send this message: I'm a captain, change course 20 degrees."

"I'm a seaman second class," came the reply. "You had better change course 20 degrees."

By that time, the captain was furious. He spat out, "Send ... 'I'm a battleship. Change course 20 degrees.'"

Back came the flashing light, "I am a lighthouse."

The captain changed course.

The captain could have chosen to disregard the truth of the lighthouse's existence, but he would have paid the price for his ignorance. It is the same with people who compulsively say, "What lighthouse? What problem? I'll just go on another diet. It'll all be OK someday." Meanwhile, they come closer and closer to a personal doomsday. That's because they keep seeing something the same way and it doesn't work—and they keep exerting their will, trying to force the problem to conform to their understanding, their picture of reality. They don't understand that what they think is a ship is really a lighthouse. The energy used for compulsive diet behavior overruns their rational thinking, and since diets are a rational approach to an irrational problem they cannot possibly work.

True change starts in the heart. I don't know of a simpler way to say it. It's the deep message of the Bible, and it's true in every part of your life. Proverbs 23:7 says, "For as he thinketh in his heart, so is he" (KJV). True change doesn't start in the head. It doesn't start in the pocketbook or with the beautician. Nagging never brought about true change. Criticism doesn't help. You cannot truly change anyone, and they cannot change you unless you're willing. No, true change only starts in one place, and that is in your heart.

That's why I'm going to suggest that you ask yourself what you want to do. Not what you think you should do and definitely not what someone else thinks you should do, but *what you want to do*. Remember when Jesus asked the crippled man who was lying by the pool in Bethesda a question: "Do you want to be healed?" (John 5:6). Jesus was not asking a rhetorical question. He wanted an answer, because Jesus knew that the answer to healing lies first in the truth within a person's heart: Do you *want* to be healed?

Now before you say to me, "But Dr. Jantz who wouldn't want to be thinner?" let me assure you that there are many different reasons for wanting to lose weight. It might be safety, anger, rebellion, fear...and the list goes on! That's why I never start out by asking someone what they eat or don't eat. That's because I have learned that the first thing that must be considered is the probability of some kind of change in a person's heart.

SOME WAYS TO START

"The God of heaven is the one who will give us success, and we his servants are going to start building."
Nehemiah 2:20

If your heart whispers, "I'm really not ready," then, perhaps, you need to work on the challenges that remain in your heart rather than work on weight management. Talk to a good friend about your fears. A counselor might be able to help. Whatever you do, don't give up. You need to start—but start at where your heart is. If, on the other hand, your heart says, "Yes, I'm ready. I want to live healthier," then I have some effective suggestions for you:

- **Limit the fat.** People who lose weight and keep it off learn the benefits of decreasing the amount of fat in their diet. One middle-aged woman who came to me,

Sally, was among that group of Americans that consumes 40 percent or more of its calories from fat. When Sally started understanding the reports of the increased risk of heart disease and cancer associated with these high levels of fat, she immediately self-corrected. She started reading labels in the supermarket and began to understand the wealth of information they contained. This was a far cry from the ineffective calorie counting and roller-coaster dieting of the past. She was now getting the kind of information she could use. She stopped frying her foods and quit breading meats. She learned that broiling, baking, and even microwave preparation were better alternatives to cooking in fats and oil.

She also started eating more lightly-steamed vegetables. Her former overweight self had also eaten vegetables, but they were "doctored" foods such as creamed corn, fried onion rings, and once-nourishing carrots now swimming in deep pools of rich butter sauce—all high in fat and cholesterol. She learned that the difference between one plain baked potato and a baked potato with "the works"—mounds of butter and gobs of sour cream—was enormous, and that she'd have to eat at least nine plain baked potatoes to equal one with all that stuff.

• **Limit refined carbs.** People who lose weight effectively learn to limit the amount of refined carbohydrates in their diet. Sally grew up with an overweight mother who loved to prepare big, fattening sack lunches for her daughter to eat at school. The sandwiches were works of art, prepared on soft slices of enriched white bread, overflowing with greasy salami, baloney (of sometimes questionable origin), and thick layers of mayonnaise and butter. Nestled in the bottom of the bag would be a *love note*, accompanied by two or three chocolate or peanut butter cookies.

Her mother may have had the best of intentions for Sally, but those good wishes later brought on disaster for a little girl now grown up, and struggling with her weight. Unwittingly, Sally's mother had played into the hands of food manufacturers who are consummate pro-

STAY CLOSE TO NATURAL

Many of the most delicious foods are naturally packed with nutrients but are unnecessarily refined to aid in their marketing and appeal. Foods such as white bread are refined to the point of losing much of their nutritional value. Stick with the unrefined stuff—the whole-grain breads and cereals—and if you're hankering for something sweet, consider a touch of molasses instead of the refined sugar in a prepackaged snack food.

fessionals when it comes to catering to our nation's taste buds. They know their science, and they know their psychology. They know we want sweet, not bland; tasty, not necessarily healthy, so they give us what they know we'll respond to. And they know we tend to respond more to pretty packages than to the all-natural, full color and richness of fruits and vegetables. They are simply good marketers, solely attendant to the bottom line. People who lose weight successfully ignore the hype, the ads, and the promotions.

• **Limit the sodas.** People who lose weight say good-bye to artificially sweetened drinks. You just don't need those sodas, diet colas, or caffeinated beverages. They do nothing but keep you dependent on still more sweets, making it virtually impossible for you to give up your addiction and move toward healthy foods. Water, water, water—it's the only alternative worth drinking. Tap water may be a risk to your health in some areas, so you may want to buy bottled water or install a water purification system in your home to make it easy for you to drink water whenever you want to. There are several good systems on the market. Water, Yes! Sodas and so-called diet drinks, nyet!

• **Eat complex carbs.** People who lose weight and keep it off eat large amounts of lightly steamed or raw vegetables, fresh fruits, and whole grains. This was a stretch for Sally at first because she and her family had never eaten this way. But over time, Sally, her husband, and their two children started to see the health benefits of this new way of eating. Today, they no longer sit down to watch television with large bags of corn chips, potato chips, or other nutrition-less, empty-calorie snack foods nestled in their laps. For them, it was a major step toward successful weight loss. Not only do these products contribute to the expanding midsection of the average American, but they are actually becoming a national health risk. It's now been determined that American families may be getting most of their refined carbohydrates during the so-called "down times" when they snack and graze on food, usually when they are bored or watching television.

Today, it's different in Sally's household. She and her family snack on raw fruits packed with nutrients; they enjoy fresh, raw vegetables without the fattening sauces and dips. While she and her children still like to go out for the occasional hamburger at fast food restaurants, it's not the norm. And even when they do go, Sally often goes for the salad bar (with lemon wedges, no high-fat dressing).

People who lose weight effectively know that complex carbohydrates are the key energy sources for the body. They eat all the fruits, vegetables, and other unre-

IF YOU'RE HUNGRY

In case this chapter has made you hungry, and I hope it has—hungry for the right kinds of foods—let me give you five practical nutritional tips:

1. If you crave something sweet after dinner, enjoy a fat-free yogurt. You'll feel better than if you had a piece of pie or a dish of ice-cream.

2. A very European supper is to eat bread and soup two to three times a week for dinner. Period! That's your main course, not a warm-up to the entree. Make it a broth- or vegetable-based soup to keep it low in calories and fat. Bon appetit.

3. If you order a rich dessert at a restaurant, split it with someone else at the table. It's automatic weight control. (And if the other person has not read this book, he or she will probably eat most of your share anyway.)

4. If you're invited to a party, enjoy one or two pieces of fruit before you go so you are not hungry when you arrive. Be full enough so that if the caterer does not appear you will not be disappointed—or famished!

5. Eliminate oils and fats when cooking. Nonfat yogurt is a good substitute for sour cream, and chicken broth used in your sauces is a sneaky—yet healthy—disguise for butter, and it's so much better for you.

fined foods they can. They reduce their consumption of refined and processed sugars. They diminish their fat consumption by reducing the amount of fatty meats they consume, and they replace foods in their diet that have saturated fats with those having unsaturated fats. They also reduce their sodium intake by decreasing the amount of salt added to their food. People who lose weight successfully enjoy eating bulky, grainy foods because they feel full for extended periods of time. Chemically, complex carbohydrates are composed of the kinds of sugars that break down much more slowly in your digestive system. This means they are absorbed more evenly into your bloodstream, keeping your energy up and your cravings down.

• **Do what Sally did.** Eat a healthy breakfast every day and reduce the amount of fat in your diet. Just start paying attention. Engage in an activity you enjoy for 15 minutes each day. The only rule is to move your body. Put your scale away. Start drinking water and eliminate sodas and diet drinks.

• **Begin a confidential journal.** In your journal or notebook, take a daily inventory about how you feel about the three deadly emotions that must be dealt with by people who lose weight successfully: anger, fear, and guilt. Don't be afraid to describe your innermost feelings. You are not writing an essay for anyone else. These are your own personal expressions, and they're critical to putting you on the track to effective weight loss. Try to write daily for one month.

If you follow the steps in this chapter, you are ready to begin changing the way you eat. It won't be a drastic change. I counsel people to run the race one step at a time rather than move out of the blocks so fast they become winded before they've begun. That's why I'm spending so much time talking about getting your heart ready to change rather than giving you a calorie-counter or a diet book. It is your heart that will help you win the race.

One Cookie for Me ... One Cookie for God

"Once when Jacob was cooking a stew, Esau came in from the field, and he was famished. Esau said to Jacob, 'Let me eat some of that red stuff, for I am famished!'...Jacob said, 'First sell me your birthright.' Esau said, 'I am about to die; of what use is a birthright to me?' Jacob said, 'Swear to me first.' So he swore to him, and sold his birthright to Jacob. Then Jacob gave Esau bread and lentil stew, and he ate and drank, and rose and went his way. Thus Esau despised his birthright."

Genesis 25:29–33

A TALE OF TWO BROTHERS

Life—I can guarantee you—is not always fair.

One of the most hotly debated stories in the Old Testament involves two brothers: Jacob and Esau.

One was beloved of his father; the other beloved of his mother. One a hunter; one a man who lived in tents. One of the brothers was to have a great promise and a great birthright, the other brother was to serve him.

This is a classic story. Esau was the eldest. The birthright belonged to him. But Jacob managed to take it away from him with little more than the smell of some good cooking. If you think it's unfair, you are right. There is little that is fair about the story, especially when it continues with trickery and deception.

Life was unfair to Esau. He was a dutiful son, and he still lost his blessing.

The reason I use this story is because I believe one of the first things we each must do in life is look around us and accept the fact that life is not always fair. You will not always get the promotion you deserve. You will not always get the praise you want. You will not always get the beauty, brains, or money that you want.

Life—I can guarantee you—is not always fair, at least not when we view it from our limited human experience. No one is cutting the pieces of pie into exactly the same sizes. Some people get more of this. Some people get more of that.

"Has God been fair to you?" The reason I ask that is because an outraged sense of fairness, and the resulting sense of envy, can be a big stumbling block to anyone who wants to live a healthier life, both physically and spiritually.

If you look at other people and say you wish you could be like they are because they're thinner or smarter or more popular, then you've not yet realized the value of your own self. Like Esau, you are giving away your birthright. What birthright? I am convinced you are wonderfully and uniquely made and that if you are doing everything you can to be the individual God created you to be, there is no one better than you on the face of the earth! That's right—no movie star, no scientist, no queen, no president.

If Esau had known the value of his own heart, soul, and person, he would not have given his birthright away for a plate of stew. There was a blessing for Esau, and Esau just gave it away. Incredible, you say?

I would agree, except I see the same thing happen time and again among people who talk with me. One day I'll talk to a man whose life is embittered because his brother became a star on the varsity football team while he, himself, was judged too uncoordinated to march in the band at half-time. This may have all taken place 20 years ago, but the man remembers it as though it were last week! The next day I'll talk to a woman who stopped speaking to her sister years ago because she felt her sister was always pointed out as the pretty one, the favored one. The sister may even be dead, and the envy continues.

In each case, envy has destroyed the person's heart. Envy makes a person's spirit shrivel up and die as surely as if that person had traded his or her birthright for a plate of stew.

Envy stops growth. Envy prevents you from being you. Instead of cultivating the flowers you're meant to have in your garden, you spend your days gazing at the flowers in someone else's garden. And why, when you have roses in your grasp, do you want orchids instead?

It's the same reason that sometimes overweight people envy every thin person they see and, instead of celebrating their own uniqueness, feel they are second-rate because they are not a size 6. The irony is that this envy does not help anyone lose weight. In fact, the opposite is usually the case.

It might sound simplistic, but it's true: Losing weight is not only about what you put in your mouth. It's about what you put in your heart and soul as well. There are "junk food" thoughts just like there are "junk food" cupcakes. These are thoughts that do not nourish us; they may look attractive, but they have no real value. Envy is high on the list of junk food thoughts.

Let's be honest. There is always going to be someone in this world—and in your life—who will be better than you are at something: better looking than you, slimmer than you, with a better personality than you, more money than you, smaller hips than you, more friends than you...and the list could go on endlessly. If you want to be miserable, live a life of making comparisons. You simply cannot win. You are who you are, and others are who they are.

THE COMPARISON TRAP

When you spend your time comparing yourself with those around you, I'm afraid at least seven challenges will emerge almost immediately:

1. You will become rigid in body and mind.
2. You will demand to be in control at all times (and, therefore, you'll find yourself out of control).
3. You will forget to smile.
4. You will dwell on what's wrong instead of what's right about you and others.
5. You will blame yourself and others for what's not going well in your life.
6. You will tend to expect the worst of yourself instead of what's best.
7. You will store your anger deep in your ever expanding gut.
8. And, most important, you will throw away God's birthright for you—the thing that makes you uniquely you!

You may not have known what to do about your envy—you may not have even named it envy. Sometimes people are so defeated they don't even know that envy keeps them down; they've turned it inside out: Instead of saying, "I envy Bev because she's so pretty," they say, "I'm ugly. I wish I were like Bev. But I'm ugly." Envy is only one side of the comparison coin—the other side is shame. That's why it's so important to celebrate who you are instead of keeping your eyes on others. Envy and shame never helped anyone lose an ounce!

THE BENIGN SIN?

"You shall not covet your neighbor's house; you shall not covet your neighbor's wife, or male or female slave, or ox, or donkey, or anything that belongs to your neighbor."
Exodus 20:17

Envy might look like no big deal, but that is only because we've become accustomed to it. We think of it as one of those "little sins" that everyone feels. But envy isn't a little sin. God thought envy was so soul-destroying that he named it in one of the Ten Commandments. To covet something is to envy someone.

By now you've probably identified some things that you may envy in others. I'd be surprised if you have not. Most of us envy others on occasion. Sometimes the envy is fleeting. But that's not the kind of envy I'm speaking of. I'm talking about the kind of envy that gets hold of you and won't give up its grip. This kind of envy can splinter families, divide marriages, separate siblings, and destroy churches. If you hold envy like this to your heart, you will weigh your soul down to the point of death.

There's only one thing to do with envy—let go of it. There's no point in trying to prove you're better than the person you envy. If you should happen to convince yourself of that fact, you will only find someone else to envy. No, the only thing to do with envy is just to let it go.

> You're not always the person you think you are, but what you think makes you the person you become.

Envy keeps you going around and around in circles, not able to move because one foot is nailed to the floor. You're frustrated because you don't seem to be getting very far in your spiritual journey; you can't move. You need to let go of envy—to have that nail removed—so you can walk along the path God has for you. Until you get rid of that nail, that stubborn envy, all you can do is walk around in an ever deepening rut.

Harold Kushner wrote, "When people are loving, brave, truthful, charitable, God is present." Robert Louis Stevenson cautioned us to "sit loosely in the saddle of life." The sentiments of these writers have been the underlying theme of my thoughts on living an emotionally healthy life. Nothing much will ever be accomplished until you cultivate and maintain a deep appreciation and love for the special person God made—you. Nor will your life have much lasting satisfaction if you do not share that love and compassion with others. This is the key to jettisoning your envy. Learn to appreciate what God has given you. Take your eyes off of others. Count your own blessings. And then share these blessings with others. The greatest blessing you have is yourself, and the greatest gift you can give to others is also yourself.

People who lose weight effectively not only "sit loosely in the saddle," they also know precisely in which direction their horse is headed. They understand that negative thoughts can rule their lives as obsessively as any addiction. That's why from this day forward you can choose to be committed to giving yourself over to expressions of hope and joy. How? Begin to turn your back on the past, and reach for forgiveness. Forgive yourself—daily if necessary—for falling short of your goals, and forgive others for any real or imagined harm they have done to you. Look at yourself in the mirror, if necessary, and say to yourself, "I forgive you for over-eating last week. I forgive you for past mistakes. I forgive you. I forgive you. I forgive you." You may feel foolish the first time you do this, but continue. Learn to speak your forgiveness.

When Jesus on the cross asked God to forgive His tormentors, He did it as much for His own peace as for the eternal soul of His tormentors. Forgiveness lightens the soul. An unforgiving heart is a heavy heart. When I speak with people who've prayed their way through to forgiveness, invariably they will say to me something like, "I feel so much better. Freer. Like a load has been lifted from me." That's because a heavy load has been lifted. Bitterness and envy are self-defeating emotions. They take up room in your heart—room that was otherwise designed to hold love, kindness, and blessings from God!

So this is a good time to stop criticizing yourself. I have never met you and still I know that if you habitually criticize yourself, you are unjustly criticizing yourself. Look beyond your faults this once. Look beyond the mistakes you've made, and instead, look at the intent of your heart. Otherwise the weight of envy, shame, and critical attitudes will weigh you down as surely as a stone around your neck.

THE GREAT STONE REMOVER

Forgiveness is a gift you can give yourself.

Forgiveness. I call it the great stone remover because it can literally lighten your heart. The foremost act that prompts us to get on with our lives, bringing pleasure to ourselves and an openhearted love to others, is forgiveness. Right now, your heart can become lighter, and you can begin to walk with your head high, with courage and confidence. It's what's destined to happen in your life as you say good-bye to the weight of envy and resentment. It may not be easy, but it is worth it.

Just how important it really is can be demonstrated in this story about a man named Paul. Without this difficult act of forgiveness, Paul would not have been able to lose weight and keep it off. In his own words:

> I HAD MUCH TO LEARN *about myself and about life. I'd been blaming others for years for my problem with weight—and, in those few seconds when I wasn't blaming someone else, I was envying them or criticizing myself. Dr. Jantz helped me understand that to intentionally forgive those who hurt me in the past*

> *would give me the permission to make the strides necessary to put my life back together. I didn't understand it at first—didn't even want to do it at first—but I needed to forgive to move toward my goal of weight loss.*

Paul is 46 years old. He grew up in a politically and religiously conservative family. Anyone observing his upbringing would probably say now there's an emotionally healthy family. They go to church, are good citizens, pay their taxes, are treated with respect in the community—they must have it made. It would be easy to make that assessment given the outward signs of emotional stability. However, there was more to the story, as there always is. Paul grew up in a family with three other brothers, all older than he. From day one Paul was treated as the baby, the last born, the one who needed to be perpetually nurtured. His mother smothered him with inappropriate care-giving as she became involved in every detail of his life. Paul was never allowed to grow up. And, even worse, he was never allowed to feel successful about anything, because any challenge was deemed too much for him. He wasn't even encouraged to do his own homework or clean his own room. Paul, it seemed, needed help with everything.

His siblings began to see him as helpless and inferior—not because he was younger, but because he was treated in ways that made him feel younger. Paul was in free fall. Emotionally handicapped, he had to find other ways to cope with his fears and self-doubts because he believed so strongly that he would never be quite good enough.

As Paul grew older, his brothers seemed to excel in everything they did, in sports, music, academics. They were the family's superstars. If awards were given, they were on stage to receive them, as their parents stood by to applaud and reward their efforts, while Paul stood in the wings wishing he could be part of the celebration.

But he was still the baby in the family—the one of whom nothing was expected and so nothing was ever achieved. Envy ate away at Paul. He saw himself as a failure at sports, at making friends, at gaining any limelight. His envy separated Paul from his brothers. He didn't like to be around them because he was constantly reminded that he wasn't as good as they were. He told himself he wasn't as smart as they were; wasn't as likable; wasn't as athletic. The truth is he could have been. But his self-defeating attitude crippled him before he tried to do anything.

Paul never even made a friend. Who would want to be friends with him, he asked? Since no friend was available, Paul quickly figured out he would have to find his own friend. He found it in the kitchen cupboard, the refrigerator, the corner store, the snack stand at the movies, in candy bars, ice cream, potato chips, in sandwiches piled high with lunch meats and drowned in dressing and mayonnaise. Paul had found food, and he made food his intimate friend. He had never learned to develop healthy relationships with his parents, his brothers, or other people. But food? That was something different. Food was readily accessible, it did not judge him, it made him feel good, and, most important, Paul felt he was finally better than everyone at something: He was better at gaining weight. And, not surprisingly, his weight finally got him the attention he wanted. His mother fussed at him, coaxing him with salads and diet pills to lose weight. Sure his brothers teased him, but at least they talked to him.

However, even with the attention, Paul was miserable. He still envied his brothers. In his heart, he knew gaining weight was not something to applaud. More than that, though, he knew deep in his heart that his extra weight only stopped him from finding something at which he could truly excel. It stopped him from being Paul. Instead, he was the "fat kid."

That's why, when Paul and I began talking, we didn't talk about food. We talked about his brothers. About his mother. About his father. Shortly after I met Paul, I asked him to make a list of the things he liked about himself. It took him 20 minutes to come up with one thing: "I make a good grilled hamburger."

We started with a grilled hamburger.

Making a grilled hamburger wasn't enough to form an identity. So I asked Paul to think of one thing he liked about himself every day for a week. At the same time, I asked him to pray for the desire to forgive his family for their treatment of him. I could not help but notice that as his prayers for forgiveness progressed and finally deepened into an actual desire to forgive, Paul found more and more things to like about himself.

> Take out a piece of paper and make a list of the things you like about yourself. They don't have to be big things; they don't have to be things others will admire—just things you like. Then tack it up in a place where you can read it every day.

Over time, Paul became more defined as a person. He found he had a dry, witty sense of humor and could make his brothers laugh. He found he was good at math and could help his mother calculate the family's taxes. Paul was no more helpless, baby Paul. And as his self-confidence grew larger and larger, his waistline grew smaller and smaller.

Paul reminded me of this spiritual truth: Envy clouds our vision. Envy separates us from God and—equally important—it separates us from the blessings God has for us. We can't cultivate the flowers in our own garden when we are hanging over the fence wishing we had the flowers in someone else's garden. We cannot truly know ourselves unless we are willing to accept the birthright God has given us, and that means making room in our hearts for the unique combination of gifts God means for us.

To discover those gifts, ask yourself: What is my dream? What good things has God given to me? What are my goals? Do I want to live a half life, complaining about my past, blaming others for my problems? Or, am I moving ahead with courage and commitment to become the person God intends? I hope your answer is, I want to accept my birthright, and I'm in charge of making it happen now!

If you can do this you are already making progress. No longer are you allowing the doubts and fears of a remote, unhealthy emotional past to keep you grounded, because you know God made you to soar on the strong wings of hope and joy. Thank God for where you've been, and then thank Him even more for where you are now and where you are going.

So Job Had Patience—I Want Results Now

"Now when Job's three friends heard of all these troubles that had come upon him, each of them set out from his home.... When they saw him from a distance, they did not recognize him, and they raised their voices and wept aloud; they tore their robes and threw dust in the air upon their heads. They sat with him on the ground seven days and seven nights, and no one spoke a word to him, for they saw that his suffering was very great."

Job 2:11–13

SEVEN DAYS OF SILENCE

Don't just do something. Sit there.

When we tell the story of Job, we usually talk about Job and his undying patience. However, every time I read his story, I'm not struck so much by Job's patience, but rather by the patience of his friends—even though they were little more than cold comfort to him at his time of need.

They were patient, yes, but they were also literal "advice machines," dispensing wisdom and giving Job reasons for his untenable condition. But as often as not, the quick fixes we offer others are for our benefit as much as for our friends. We, ourselves, seem to be the ones who are uncomfortable with unresolved problems.

Some people say that we need to see our problems resolved in 30 minutes or less because that's the length of the average television show. That may be true, but I think we may expect quick fixes because we don't want to do like Job's friends—we don't want to sit with our problems—or anyone else's. Sitting makes us nervous. It reminds us there may be nothing we can do. We feel

> Sometimes sitting with our problems is the best thing we can do. Quick fixes can make things worse. Sometimes the long way around a problem is the only way around it.

powerless and, therefore, impatient. Even our prayers are often filled with spoken, or unspoken, deadlines: "God, please do such-and-such and do it *now!*"

The reason I point out the importance of patience to people is because almost everyone I counsel eventually reaches the point where they are exasperated with how long a process healthy weight loss is. Notice that I said *healthy* weight loss; extreme diets promise dramatic weight loss, but this is never healthy. Diet ads seduce you with promises of quick fixes; don't be deceived. Your body needs time to lose the weight so that it's fat you lose and not muscle or water. Weight that comes off quickly goes back on even quicker and usually brings a few more pounds with it to keep it company.

GOOD THINGS TAKE TIME

"The testing of your faith produces endurance; and let endurance have its full effect, so that you may be mature and complete, lacking in nothing."
James 1:3–4

Building a healthy body is like building a healthy soul. It takes time. The older I grow, the more I realize that character comes from experience, and experience comes from time. The bark of an older tree is more interesting than that of a young sapling. The goals we value most in life are the goals that require time and effort. There are no magic wands that bring meaningful, instant success. This is especially true when it comes to building a healthier body.

Some months ago I received a letter from a woman I'll call Connie. Connie had come to see me almost a year ago looking for a quick way to lose weight before her daughter's wedding. She pressed me on how long it would take her to lose 60 pounds, adding that she'd seen a diet plan that would show her how to lose it in two months. "Could I do that?" she asked hopefully. That would make her slim just in time for the wedding. When I told her two months was not enough time to lose that amount of weight in a healthy manner, she left. I did not think I would ever hear from her again, but then I got this letter.

> Have you ever noticed that some people take better care of their cars than they do of their bodies—regular mainte-nance, good-quality fuel, preventive repairs—and yet they'll own several cars in their lifetime while they'll only have one body in this life.

DEAR DR. JANTZ: *Remember me. I was the impatient one. I wanted to write and let you know that I didn't take your advice. I dove right into that diet plan with those diet pills. Only $9.95 for a week's supply. What a deal! At first it seemed like it was going to work. The pounds were melting off—or so I thought.*

Then I began to think it wasn't the pounds that were melting, but that it was me melting away. I started having nightmares. I couldn't concentrate at work. I told myself it was all the excitement about the wedding, but I didn't really believe it. Finally, I stopped the pills. I'd lost 30 pounds and decided that would be enough. I bought a new "mother of the bride" dress. I was proud of myself. But then the weight started coming back. And I wasn't eating that much—even less than I used to! One day I didn't eat anything but a salad with lemon juice and a banana and I still gained a pound! I couldn't believe it. My daughter hadn't even returned from her honeymoon before the scale notched up ten pounds. Before I knew it, I was right back where I started—and then some! Can I come back and try again?

I called Connie. She came in to see me shortly after that, and we did begin again. The first thing she did was put a sign on her refrigerator door that said, "You can build a new life—one day at a time." Every time she feels impatient, she looks at that sign. We remind each other that steady progress is the key to taking weight off—and keeping it off!

Connie's sign belongs on more than a refrigerator. I am convinced that one very important key to a satisfying spiritual life is patience. To pray requires patience. God usually does not answer instantaneously—or even within the same week! The Bible tells us that as we mature, God expects us to develop more patience in our lives. The Letter of James says, "the testing of your faith produces endurance; and let endurance have its full effect, so that you may be mature and complete, lacking in nothing" (James 1:3–4).

Notice how endurance, or patience, is tied with the phrase "lacking in nothing." Patience grows into contentment. Sometimes the things we want so desperately at the moment are not what we really want in the long run. Waiting, in this case, lets us separate our fleeting fancies and passing whims from the deep and true desires of our heart. As anyone with a young child can tell you, teaching patience is one of the best ways to build character. If you were to give in to every desire of a two-year-old instantaneously, the child would never grow in character.

I am spending the time to talk about patience because we often think of patience and waiting as an empty time—a time of doing nothing. But waiting can be a very important, even critical, time in our development. That's why, even though I counsel patience to anyone working on a weight-loss program, I emphasize that it is not just for our bodies' sake that we learn the art of patience.

Patience benefits our souls as much as it ever does our bodies. Remember, the Apostle Paul charged us to "run with perseverance the race that is set before us" (Hebrews 12:1). Even in the midst of running a race, patience is the key. Without patience, endurance, and perseverance, discouragement sets in. And with discouragement comes defeat. Patience is not a passive time. Patience is a time of growing.

I'm not advocating passive patience. On the contrary, I'm encouraging active patience—patience that comes with taking the first step in the direction you know you need to go—perseverance. Paul didn't say to "sit on the sidelines with your patience." He clearly said to join the race.

When you decide to lose weight and develop a healthier physical body, you have chosen a direction. You know where you want to go. You have joined the race. Patience will help you get to the goal line because it will help you put one foot in front of the other at a steady pace instead of sprinting out fast, wearing yourself out, and not finishing the race. Walking down any spiritual or physical path requires patience—the spiritual path to weight loss is no exception.

When I think of all the people riding the "diet cycle," I realize how important patience is. These are the men and women—and increasingly the children—who gain and lose the same 20 pounds every six months throughout their lives. They treat their bodies like a yo-yo, up and down, and then up and down again.

CONSIDER THESE STATISTICS

- 44 percent of high school girls, and 15 percent of high school boys reported they were trying to lose weight.
- 50 percent of adult women and 24 percent of adult men are on a diet on any given occasion.
- It's estimated that 10 percent of Americans (25 million people) have disordered eating.

We all know that as a nation we have a serious problem. It's estimated that one in three Americans is overweight, an increase of 30 percent in the last ten years. Still, when we hear these statistics, we somehow are still tempted to rush out and do something—invent yet another diet; start a government program or a television campaign. The truth is that the problem will take time to resolve, and we will remain defeated in our attempts to solve the problem unless we demonstrate patience. Quick weight loss is not effective weight loss. The only thing this impatience leads to is eating disorders.

YOU'VE GOT TIME

"For everything there is a season, and a time for
every matter under heaven."
Ecclesiastes 3:1

One bright, sunny day a young farm boy ran up to his granddad who was returning from the field. "Grandpa, quick, tell me, how much time do I have?"

Granddad answered simply, "You have just enough time, son."

"But how much time will it take for me to be big and grown up like you?" the boy asked, tugging on his Grandpa's pant's leg.

The old man smiled, "Just like everything else, my boy, it will take just the right amount of time."

"Why do I have to be a boy? Why do I have to wait so long? Why can't I just be a man like you?" the boy asked, frustration now filling his young, tender face.

Grandpa knelt down and looked his grandson straight in the eye, saying, "Son, when you do one thing right—at the right time—the next thing works even better, and you, one day, will become what you want to become."

Time is your most precious asset. To think otherwise can lead you to overwhelming regret, frustration, and even despair. Even though we may not speak of it much in this book, these pages are actually all about time—about the critical 24 hours a day and the 168 hours each week you have to choose your direction in life. I'd love to be able to give you more time to help you accelerate the speed of your spiritual and emotional growth that will propel you to effective weight loss, but that would be physically impossible. I just can't give you that gift of extra time. But you don't need any more time. You already have all the time you need.

YOU'VE ALREADY TAKEN THE FIRST STEP

In the challenge to reach your goals, there is only one way to move: forward.

You've already taken that all-important first step in your plan by taking your first steps down the path. I would imagine you chose this book for one primary reason: You want to lose weight and have a healthier physical life. Be assured, you have chosen the right book because in these pages we aren't talking about diets or any other form of extreme weight management behavior. People who lose weight and keep it off don't need to be extreme.

People who follow a spiritual path to weight loss know they need patience. Patience keeps them steady.

They can jump into the same water as they did before but this time the tide does not sweep them away. There is no swimming against the current, no ineffective paddling upstream, fearing that drowning is imminent. People who lose weight with patience, work with and cooperate with the current. They do not resist it. Diets and programs of self-deprivation teach you to set up a resistance to growth, which is the opposite result you are seeking. The unfortunate truth is that dieting can establish a pattern of eating disorders that often persists for a lifetime.

That's why I've written this chapter—to help keep you from sabotaging the successes you'll have as you start your spiritual path to weight loss. Now is the time to close the chapter on your ineffective past and open a new chapter that will lead to your better, brighter future.

The future may seem uncertain now. That is why I want to assure you that you are not the only one to have walked down the spiritual path to weight loss. Sometimes people tell me they can't even walk, they crawl down that path. Slowly. Inch by inch. They have shared their stories with me over the years and I have made some observations about those who are successful in losing weight:

• **People who successfully lose weight know they're not alone in the struggle.** They quickly discover they are not islands of pain in an ocean of happiness. Pain is everywhere. No one is immune to sadness or grief. Everyone carries a burden—a cross. Just as important, people who lose weight effectively learn there are many who are ready, willing, and able to empathize with them and work at understanding what they are going through.

• **People who successfully lose weight admit they have a need to be accepted.** To be accepted means to be taken seriously—something that usually does not happen to us when we're young. People who lose weight effectively learn to ask for what they need, because they know if they don't get what they need—acceptance—they will head to the refrigerator to get what they think they need—a piece of pie, a cupcake, a bowl of ice cream.

• **People who successfully lose weight know they need to have someone affirm them.** We all need to know that the character we play on the stage of life has significance, and that we are here for a purpose. Nothing is more painful than to be unnoticed, unrecognized, and unaffirmed. People who lose weight effectively learn the amazing truth that they are important—an importance that has nothing to do with the size of their clothing or where they are on the journey to weight loss. For Christians, God has given us a special sign of our importance: He loves and transforms us daily.

A warm relationship with God can be the bedrock of a successful weight-loss program. The spiritual path to weight loss is a sure path. That's why, in the next section of this book, we will spend time talking about our relationship with the Creator as it relates to weight loss. We will talk about the God who made us who we are, and who is re-shaping us every day.

> You are growing an oak, not a sunflower. One takes years; the other a few dog days of summer. Long after the seasons have sent the sunflower packing, the oak continues to put its roots deeper into the ground because it knows it's been designed for the long haul. It endures the rigors of the environment and the challenges that growth demands because the mighty oak has a plan for its better future—just as you have a plan for yours.

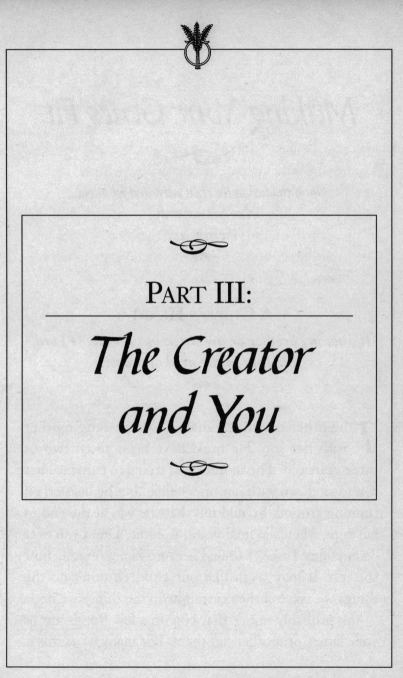

PART III:

The Creator and You

Making Your Genes Fit

"Train children in the right way, and when old,
they will not stray."
Proverbs 22:6

A CHILD'S HEART

*It's not my brother or my sister, but it's me, O Lord,
standing in the need of prayer.*

The other day in the mall, I saw a young mother with her son. He must have been about two or three years old. The mother was trying to convince her son to sit down with her on a bench, but he insisted on running around. I could tell that she was at the end of her rope when she finally said to him, "Don't you ever do anything I ask?" I smiled because I knew exactly how she felt. It may seem like our children don't do the things we ask, but they certainly do the things we do.

You probably notice that you do a few things just as your father or mother did them. For many of us this is not bad. But for others, the habits we learned in our family haunt us, sometimes almost drive us crazy.

I have some liberating news for you: You do not need to continue bad patterns from your childhood. That's right. You do not need to continue along that same road. The first step to changing those old patterns of behavior is to recognize that you *can* change them. You may have been told it was your upbringing that made you overweight. You couldn't help it, you lived on a farm and all the family ate was meat, potatoes, and apple pie à la mode. But you are no longer a child. The choices you make today are freely made.

Of course our early environment plays a role in every area of our lives. Our genetic make-up is also a factor. If you have reason to believe that genetics—your DNA— is the reason you are overweight, then you may need to consult a medical doctor. You may, indeed, have a physical problem. However, for most of us, the family weight problems we inherited are problems related to the lifting of the fork and what we place on that fork.

You may be telling yourself you're an overeater because that's just the way it's done in your family—after all, look at the size of Uncle Bob and Grandma Mary. The time to stop this line of thinking is now, because this may have all the hallmarks of an excuse. Worse than just being an excuse, it can keep you stuck in a dangerous rut. People who lose weight and keep it off move beyond blaming others for their weight challenges. They take responsibility for their own actions because they know it's the only way they will ever grow into the person God created them to be.

People who lose weight effectively also learn to take full responsibility for their own emotional state of being. Blaming family is taking the easy way out, and it's a dead-end street. Perhaps the theme song of those who lose weight successfully should be the great spiritual that reminds us, "It's not my brother or my sister, but it's me, O Lord, standing in the need of prayer. Yes, Lord, it's me." And it's you. The buck stops here.

WHOSE SHOES?

Seen in a church bulletin: "Shoes divide people into three classes. Some wear their father or mother's shoes, and they make no declaration of their own. Some are unthinkingly shod by the crowd. But the really strong people are those who are their own cobbler, insisting on making their own choices. These are the ones who walk in their own shoes."

BREAKING FOOD HABITS

Bad habits are like comfortable beds; easy to get into, but hard to get out of.

~

I know how hard it is to break food habits that have grown up with you over the years. Believe me, it's just as hard to break any habit of long-standing. But sometimes these habits have to go before we can begin the spiritual path to a better, healthier new life. This is true not only of weight loss, but of almost any goal worth achieving. When you're first looking down this path, it may seem as if your goal is a distant, hazy landmark far, far away. But don't afflict yourself with unnecessary worry.

You don't need to arrive at the end of your journey with your first hesitant step. So don't focus on how difficult the next 12, 15, or even 100 steps will be. All you need to be concerned about right now is that one step in the right direction, and I know that you can take that one step, because it's that one step that gives you the power to take the next one.

People who lose weight successfully do not spend their hours worrying and complaining about their powerlessness to cope with the challenges of weight management. That's nothing but a distraction. Simply focus on taking that first step. Pretend you're a horse with blinders, whose attention is constantly being kept on the path at hand, unable to see either to the right or left. First step. Second step. That's all the horse needs to know. That's all you need to know, too. Guard your ears as well as your eyes. Don't allow anyone to say or imply that you have no power, that you will never be able to reach the end of the path so there's no sense in even beginning your journey. Of course you have power, and plenty of it.

Why does it work? Because quite the opposite of those wallowing in the mire of powerlessness, people who lose weight and keep it off learn to regain and reassert their personal power. They start to engage in a healthy self-focus, but do not fall into narcissism. To become intimately acquainted with your deepest troubles and hurts is the process of self-knowledge that allows you to look at your own soul with tender compassion, something you may not have done for some time.

In the process, you learn that you do have a power given to you by your heavenly Father, and that even the *thought* of "powerlessness" for you has now become an alien idea. The Bible talks about that power. St. Paul reminds us, "I can do all things through Him who strengthens me"(Philippians 4:13). *All things* includes living a healthier life. *All things* includes putting some of the problems that contribute to your desire to overeat behind you. *All things* includes starting down that spiritual path to weight loss.

MY DAUGHTER THE ATHLETE—PLEASE!

No one who truly loves you wants you to be someone you're not.

~·~

I'll call her Kimberly. She loved her father, but she never believed her father loved or accepted her. The reason was simple. Her father hoped against hope that Kimberly would one day become a famous athlete. Her father had wanted to be a star athlete himself, but a knee injury stopped him. Now he was intent that nothing stop Kimberly.

There was only one problem: Kimberly didn't want to become an athlete. In fact, she wasn't that well coordinated, didn't have much speed, and got more enjoyment just being a spectator. But that didn't stop her father. He made Kimberly join the softball, volleyball, and basketball teams. He would take her to the local park and they'd kick soccer balls, hit softballs, run laps, take tennis lessons—all to the point of obsession.

There was seldom a night when Kimberly did not go to bed in tears. "Dad, I don't want to become an athlete. I hate it. I love you and want to please you, but why do you want me to be someone I'm not. Why don't you like me for being me? Why are you making me do all these things I don't want to do?"

Before long, Kimberly gravitated to food as her only real source of comfort. The love and acceptance she could not get from her father was available in the refrigerator, in high-fat candy bars, in half-gallons of ice cream, and at the local bakery where she became a regular patron each day after school. Before long, Kim ballooned in weight—until she was so large that she could not go to the park anymore with her father. Every movement took her breath away. She could hardly walk anymore, much less run. Finally, she had found a legitimate excuse for not performing on the field. Kimberly found a way to put distance between herself and her father's expectations.

Even though the agony of overweight and displeasure with herself was painful, it provided relief from the relentless expectations of her father. Her father finally gave up, although his disappointment hung over them like a cloud. So she avoided her father as much as she could. Obsession with food became her substitute for fatherly affection and the neutral nondemanding love object she craved. Unfortunately, her father never dealt with his own pathology and continued to berate his daughter for not becoming the person she should have become (that is, not becoming the person he envisioned his daughter to be).

The happy part of this story is that many years later Kimberly came to The Center where our staff of counselors worked with her for several months. She recognizes she may never have the privilege of enjoying the fatherly love she'd always craved, but she also knows that what she missed is no longer a viable adult excuse for remaining overweight. Kimberly has forgiven her obsessive father, and she is getting on with her life. Her father will probably never realize it, but Kimberly won a bigger victory by doing that than she ever could have on the sport's field.

No more self-sabotaging behavior for Kimberly, and no more sneak attacks as she now enters adulthood as a growing, emotionally healthy individual. It has not been easy for her, nor will it necessarily be easy for you. Please remember that you will never completely arrive. Life will always be filled with challenges—some so great you'll wonder if you'll ever meet them.

So with that awareness, I encourage you to step out and face your fears. Keep on discovering who you are, what you want, and how you plan to get there. Determine not to miss out on the real pleasures and the real lessons of life.

You, too, may have felt pressured as a child to be someone you weren't. Athletic events are one prize, but many children are also pressured to be popular or superstars in the classroom. The unrealistic expectations of your family may have caused you, too, to turn to food as a comfort and a way to avoid other challenges.

FAMILY FOOD PROBLEMS

The family that eats together, gains together.

Let's look at some of the areas where these self-sabotaging behaviors may have begun. First, some questions about your father that may provide insight into your present situation:

- Did your father sabotage you in any way as a child?
- Did he always refer to the women in your home as "girls" no matter how old they were?
- Did he tend to show you a lack of respect?
- Was it a macho household where your father ruled with an iron fist?
- How did your father treat the women in your home in general?

- If you are a man, and as a child weren't aggressive, did your father infer that you might be weak, a wimp, or just a boy—regardless of your age?

- Was there an unwritten rule that suggested that women were essentially powerless?

- Did you grow up in a home where your father never cooked a meal and didn't even know how to use the washer or dryer—and only dried dishes when guests came who could see him in the kitchen at work?

- Did you grow up in a home where women were expected to do everything?

- What were the male/female generational patterns that taught you to be unhappy with yourself?

- Were men in your family viewed as the "full vessel" whereas women were "half vessels?"

The questions could go on indefinitely, but here's what I'm getting at: If you grew up in a home where the men—father, brothers, uncles—had all the answers, then you were raised in an environment where there was great risk for weight gain as a way of coping with your stress, even though the anxiety may have been unconscious. What were your other choices? Not many. You didn't throw bricks through the windows, you didn't quit bathing or engage in other socially unacceptable behaviors, but you did begin to gain weight. You probably said, hey, everyone has to eat, and it sure feels good to me. In fact, food feels like a great friend. So you ate, and ate, and ate, and ate.

This form of self-help was little more than an alternative "medicine" for something we either do not understand or do not even know exists. However, excessive eating only further aggravates the symptoms and makes the patient sicker, more despondent, often to the point of despair. Earlier I spoke of not blaming your family for your problem of overweight, but rather accepting your home environment as a fact of your early life, like it or not, appreciate it or not. Research now tells us that our food patterns for life are set around the age of five. But like anything else, you can change those patterns as an adult and start enjoying the exciting journey of becoming the person—the individual person—you desire to be.

Therefore, if you can gain a clearer perspective on what happened in your youthful past, you will be in a better position to join the ranks of those who lose weight successfully. This is because awareness is the first step toward your better emotional health and brighter future.

How can you gain that perspective? I often suggest to people that they do some of the following exercises to help them remember and understand eating patterns in their family:

• Draw a picture of your kitchen table and then mark the various places where you and the other members of your family sat when you were a child. Go back in time and recreate some of your earliest conversations with your parents, brothers, and sisters. What was said? Who said it? Were you the oldest, youngest? What was mealtime like for you as a youngster?

• If you have a family recipe book, go through it and look at the recipes. What kinds of foods did your family eat and why? Who made the food choices and planned menus in your family?

• Talk to an aunt or sister about what food meant to your family. How did your family celebrate? Was food a way of keeping in touch with your culture? Was it considered "polite" to eat a lot? Were you pressured to eat to please the cook? Was food a reward or a consolation?

The answers to all of these questions will help you understand what food meant to your family. We've all heard the coaxing that goes on in some families: "You don't like the stuffing? Please, eat the stuffing. Aunt Mary made it especially for you." Sometimes changing one's food habits means challenging your whole family's way of eating. The odd thing is that, in my conversations with people, I find that many of them report eating in the family style even when the family is hundreds of miles away. These family habits can be changed.

However, not all of our family and food-related problems have to do with habits. Some of them are much deeper problems and, because of this, I'm taking the next chapter to focus on them. I know from years of clinical experience that you, too, may have been part of a family that helped push you into using food to comfort your soul when you were only a child. Please take time to read the next chapter so you'll be better prepared to face your unique challenges.

From Daddy's Little Princess to Nobody's Queen

"But before they lay down, the men of the city, the men of Sodom, both young and old, all the people to the last man, surrounded the house, and they called to Lot, 'Where are the men who came to you tonight? Bring them out to us, that we may know them.' Lot went out of the door to the men, shut the door after him, and said, 'I beg you, my brothers, do not act so wickedly. Behold, I have two daughters who have not known man; let me bring them out to you, and do to them as you please; only do nothing to these men, for they have come under the shelter of my roof.'"

Genesis 19:4–8

I'm uncomfortable every time I read the above section of scripture. You probably are, too. This is in the Bible?! Parents are supposed to protect their children, not throw them to the wolves. We all believe this in our hearts. It's one of the basic beliefs we hold first as children and then as adults. But the sad truth is that not all parents can be trusted. The story of Lot's betrayal of his daughters could come from today's headlines instead of an account written thousands of years ago. Parents who abuse their children—who betray the trust their children have in them—have lived on this earth for a long time.

Over the years, I have spoken with many children—often grown children in their 40s or 50s—who are still damaged by the abuse and betrayal of their fathers, their mothers, or other important people in their past. Perhaps you are such a child, still in pain no matter what your age. This chapter is certainly not for everyone, but many of us live daily with the repercussions of a less-than-healthy childhood. If you suspect that your eating habits (or overeating habits) may stem from more than a sweet tooth, or even if you're not sure why you have that sweet tooth, read on and see if any of this sounds familiar.

VICTIM NO MORE

Why is it some parents treat strangers with more kindness than their own children?

It's coming to light that many who have weight challenges have been abused in one way or another in the past. Not all people, of course, but a significant number. You may be such a person, and yet, you may have

HAVE YOU EVER BEEN TOLD...

- you were stupid, and that you'd never amount to anything, no matter how hard you tried?
- your sister was prettier than you? your brother was smarter than you? your classmates did better work than you?
- you were lazy and God help you if you turn out to be like your father, or mother, or uncle, or aunt?

Do any of these questions fit? If so, you have been an unwitting victim of faulty past programming, which is, at its very least, a form of emotional abuse. As a child, if someone said you were ugly, or dumb, or not as smart as someone else, your brain believed it—even if you knew it was not true. Left unresolved, those thoughts festered, became deeply ingrained in your subconscious, and eventually became so much a part of your development that they literally ruled your life.

never dealt with the issue because of the emotional trauma you feared it might release. It's frightening to acknowledge that our parents or caretakers never took good care of us.

However, I encourage you to take a look at your past and be as honest as you can with yourself. If the word abuse is too strong, or even inappropriate for you, then I would like you to substitute the word victimization, because most weight problems have as their backdrop some form of victimization. You may have suffered emotional put downs, physical beatings, sexual assaults, perpetual rudeness by a family member, or lack of moral support—the "You'll never amount to anything" kind of statements that can create scars to last a lifetime. All those feelings you still have about those events will have an effect on how you view food.

That's why it's important for you to relive them momentarily, even if it's painful to do so.

To help you understand what I mean, let me list for you some of the characteristics of people who develop food-related problems:

• They often grew up as a perfectionist (high expectations from father, either verbalized or not; often first born).

• Their mother has a history of dieting (overemphasis on weight and appearance).

• They grew up in a home where father was "emotionally distant" (desire to please father; unsuccessful attempts to gain father's approval).

• They often had a mother who was a co-dependent (father may have been an alcoholic or addict).

• They had homes with overly strict discipline, where punishment was severe and physical.

• They had parents who used guilt and shame to discipline or punish.

• They had homes in which sexuality was not discussed, or considered "dirty."

• They had homes in which children were forced to be adults (daughters who "raised" other kids and were not allowed to be children themselves).

• They may have been sexually abused.

• They were victims of any type—victims of neglect or verbal abuse.

• There were addictions in the home. Compulsive dieting, fasting, or diuretic use; laxative abuse; prescription drug abuse.

• They have a desire to overplease others (overcontrol through people-pleasing).

• They have a tendency to ignore or deny anger.

• They overuse food for pleasure or reward (food becomes the primary focus for pleasure or to self-medicate).

LINDA'S STORY

*She knew God had given her a higher purpose for
living, and one of those purposes was to get in touch
with her big, loving heart and take the chance of
getting close to people, even though the thought still
scared her to death.*

When I gave this list to one of my overweight friends
(I'll call her Linda), she was able to relate to every issue
presented in the above chart—from perfectionism, to a
distant father, to a mother hooked on diets, to an
intense desire to hide her own feelings by overpleasing
others. Mixed within these childhood traumas, she had
also had many troubling issues during puberty where
boys made fun of her body, her height, her complexion,
and her large breasts. High school was a nightmare for
Linda. But the more she hid her emotions, the larger
she became. By the time she left school, Linda weighed
180 pounds.

When I had her write down her story, these are some
of the words she had to say:

> I REMEMBER DAYS *when I cried myself to sleep
> and woke up the next morning with tears in
> my eyes. I felt like I didn't have a friend in the*

*world. I had no one to talk to—my mother just
got upset if I tried to talk to her, and my
father...well, I didn't even try to talk to him.
I used to fantasize about what my life would be
like if I only had parents who cared about me.
I even used to pretend that I was adopted and
my real mother and father would come for me
one day. But they never did. I was so unhappy
during those years, I'm surprised I made it
through them.*

During that time, Linda never experienced any sexual or physical abuse. No one ever touched her inappropriately, but the emotional abuse she suffered was more than she could bear without the help of food. The emotional pain of unresolved anger and resentment may stem from

• the sense that you've been treated unfairly.

• the sure knowledge that no matter how hard you tried, it never made any difference.

• the terrible fear that it was really all your fault they treated you that way.

• the debilitating realization you were an idiot to think and hope that someday they'd change.

Linda eventually expressed some of these feelings as she slowly emerged from a learned helplessness to what she called a tiny flicker of hope. She was no longer willing to use the inner space of her heart to store garbage from the past. She knew God had given her a higher purpose for living, and one of those purposes was to get in touch with her big, loving heart and take the chance of getting close to people, even though the thought still scared her to death.

The first thing Linda told me after she came to this decision, however, was that she didn't know how to be close to people. She'd spent her life hiding from people. She needed help in learning how to be intimate.

TIPS FOR BUILDING INTIMACY

You can't learn to swim by reading a book, and you will never achieve intimacy with others unless you take the risk of being in their presence.

First, if your wounds do not receive proper attention, they will get worse, not better. If you have deep emotional scars get help, either from a caring pastor, professional counselor, or someone else whom you trust. Learn to see what life is around you. If you have lived many years in denial of problems, you will need to increase your awareness of what is happening around you. You may have had people trying to flag you down for friendship over the years and you didn't even notice.

Second, to become closer to other people, you must take the high dive—intentionally putting yourself in the company of a variety of people, difficult though it may be. It could be a small Bible study, a support or therapy group, a community project, a fellowship group; the choice is yours, but choose something to join now. There's a saying that you can't get to first base without leaving home plate behind. It's the same with the challenge you face in moving closer to others. Move quietly away from your past isolation and get involved at the most basic level with other people. Even if you do not participate fully in the event, at least be there quietly to demonstrate your new strength by having the courage to be present.

> "There are friends who pretend to be friends, but there is a friend who sticks closer than a brother" (Proverbs 18:24). Seek to be, and to find, such a friend and Him from whom all friends proceed.

Third, I urge you to come to grips with the kinds of people who are a challenge to you—individuals who trouble you or seem to make you feel uncomfortable, self-conscious, and ill-at-ease. Who are these people in your life? Are they neighbors, relatives, a boss? If you are a woman and are uncomfortable around men, put yourself in the presence of "safe" men where you can practice being the kind of person you are becoming without losing your personal power or your own unique identity.

Fourth, survey your past. Look at those relationships that have involved conflict, hurt, and pain. You may have been the recipient of the hurt, or you may have been the giver. Whichever, look at the conflict squarely and determine to do something redemptive. People who lose weight successfully learn to do this on a regular basis. They see and feel the hurt, and they forgive. This person may have hurt you in the meanest way, and you may want him or her to suffer even more than you. Such an attitude is understandable but not acceptable if you are committed to ongoing emotional growth. If you would be whole, you must take the chance of the high dive of forgiveness, the risk of being made a fool of, of not being understood, of swallowing your pride for your own emotional and physical health because there is simply no other way to become the whole person you say you want to be.

Fifth, to make an immediate shift in your ability to get closer to others, select two or three people you work with, live with, or come in close contact with on a regular basis. Write down three ways you would like to see

SEVENTY TIMES SEVEN

To move down the spiritual path toward successful weight loss, you must begin to empty the storage tank of emotional toxins and past resentments that are making you sick, and keeping you fat. Do you remember when Peter asked Jesus, "Lord, how often will my brother sin against me, and I forgive him? Up to seven times?" Jesus answered, "I tell you not up to seven times, but up to seventy times seven." The point was not to forgive 490 times, but to forgive, and forgive, and forgive, and then to keep on forgiving. That was wisdom of 2,000 years ago. The guiding principle has not changed.

your relationship with them improve. Then, begin to work on enriching and enhancing that relationship. Because you have been a food addict, you may have assembled a group of codependents who have not been honest with you about what they knew was going on in your life. Now is your opportunity to take the offensive with your new awareness and begin to effect positive changes in your relationships with others. Be aware that your former compulsive, obsessive eating has also made a great impact on others, but now you have started to shift your thinking. You now understand that people who lose weight and keep it off recognize that real love for others starts with a deep compassion and love for themselves. Ill health has just as much a ripple effect as emotionally healthy behavior. As you change, become closer to others. Make a consistent effort to re-adjust, even when it creates pain and possible misunderstanding. But those who lose weight for the long term know it is worth the risk of the high dive—making the first move towards emotional health. Choose a few people with whom you want more honest, healthier relationships. Then begin to use the principles in this book to help bring your objectives into reality.

Sixth, those who succeed on the spiritual path to weight loss know they must become healthy problem-solvers and bridge-builders for past relationships that have fallen on hard times. They understand that we were never made to go it alone. That no man or woman is an island. That deep within the person with a weight problem is a big, loving heart that desperately wants to touch someone, hug someone, love someone, and be touched and loved in return. The good news is that there is *always* hope. You may have been hurt beyond measure, embarrassed, shamed, made to feel guilty, and damaged emotionally. You may be off the scale when it comes to anger. But please never forget: The damage is not permanent. You are becoming free to be authentic again.

No longer do you need to allow your addictions, unresolved anger, compulsions, or obsessions to hide your big, loving heart. Starting now, you have more than enough information to begin your new life and to move toward your better future. Look for emotionally creative ways to solve your problems. Find a broken bridge, and with God's help and your new insights into who you are, attempt to rebuild a relationship that may have fallen on hard times because of unresolved anger. It's what those who lose weight do today, tomorrow, and for the rest of their lives.

> It's easy to be discouraged about weight loss. That's why I tell people to remember the woodpecker. He owes his success to the fact that he keeps pecking away until he finishes the job.

ALL FAMILIES HAVE SHADOWS

You really are free to become the person God created you to be.

No family is perfect. If there were a perfect family, the moment you and I were to enter it, it would no longer be perfect, because we would bring with us our own imperfections. Out of the many imperfections comes the family's shadows that contain secrets perhaps kept locked up for as many as two or three generations. It is these secrets, and the pain they hold in the shadows of our past, that may have gone unnoticed and may even be unknown to you now. But until you take the high dive and look at what's difficult to look at, you may continue to suffer from the stress of it and find yourself living out the symptoms of that stress—symptoms such as panic, anxiety attacks, chronic irritability, potential fear to the point of terror, sleep disorders, flashbacks, withdrawal, isolation, depression, chronic feelings of helplessness, hyper vigilance (extreme nervousness or worry), intimacy dysfunction, and other psychosomatic illnesses that have lives of their own.

The good news is that you have endured this trauma and are still alive. That means there's still hope. You've made it this far. You could have engaged in more severe, radical self-destructive behavior, but you did not. You simply chose to adjust your life with the only way you knew how to cope, through overeating and a serious affair with food. Although it continues to cause you pain, you have not given up hope. Now, since you are learning to be your own parent, you have the responsibility and the privilege of repairing yourself. You can do it now because you are an adult. You couldn't do it as a child. Times have changed. More important, you have changed. Hope is now within your grasp. This means you no longer need to punish yourself with destructive behavior. You can give it up. It's no longer you. You really are free to become the person God created you to be.

You no longer need to deny your past. You are learning that you have the courage to face what happened early in your life, recognize that's not who or what you are today, and press on to begin the spiritual path to weight loss. Denial protected you so you could keep being destructive to yourself. That is no longer an option for you. The denial of the past has served its purpose (even though it was ineffective): to keep your damaged self-esteem in check and to prevent it from being overwhelmed. Hiding from your past has kept you toxic and has assured you that you'll remain in bondage. Now you no longer need to hide from their past, troublesome and fearful though it may have been.

God made you great and wonderful. You are His child, and created in His image. You have enormous value. Now, perhaps for the first time, you are beginning to see and feel it. That's why we say people with compulsive behaviors have great, big, loving hearts. It's there. We just need to find it. As I said earlier, this may have been a difficult chapter for you to read. In fact, even as you read this page you may be recalling past events that are triggering old ways of response. If so, I urge you to talk to a counselor who will understand you as a whole person, and will help you now. Meanwhile, keep taking the occasional backward glance to your past, for in that search, you will find some of the reasons for your present challenges.

But don't delay. It's time to face your challenges head-on. If you choose not to, your compulsive behavior—primary or secondary—could remain an infected wound that may never heal. By medicating yourself with food you may have thought you were engaged in a healing process, but you have been going about it in a way that will never yield the results you desire. Overeating, secretive living, an obsession with television, hiding food, lying, and whatever behaviors you may be engaging in, might seem innocent enough. In fact, they are an anchor on your body and a tether to your soul, dragging you to places you do not wish to go.

She Eats Like a Bird

"*Stolen waters are sweet, and bread eaten in
secret is pleasant.*"
Proverbs 9:17

SECRET, SECRET, WHO'S GOT A SECRET?

*Sin boldly if you're going to sin. It's the sin that's
carefully hidden that kills a person's soul more readily
than the one that is aired for anyone to see.*

I seldom talk about food with people at first, but sometimes a person who comes to see me will say they
themselves don't have a problem with food—that they
eat like a bird and they just don't understand what's
wrong. That's when I ask them, "Do you have any food
that is hidden in your house, or car, or desk, or purse?"
There was a time when I wouldn't have thought this was
an important question. What's a little secret hoard of
food, I reasoned. But I was wrong. Keeping food hidden is one test of the depths of a person's addiction to

food, and it can be one of the greatest stumbling blocks to those who want to walk down the spiritual path of weight loss.

Chronic secrets almost always spell trouble. Secrets are a form of denial. "No, really, I couldn't eat another bite. That salad was plenty." Of course it was; you'd already eaten a chocolate bar and a bag of M&M's candy that you thought somehow didn't count because no one knew about it but you! The courage to live openly—whether it be eating openly or sinning openly—is a pre-requisite for change. The Protestant reformer Martin Luther advised people to sin boldly if they were going to sin. It's the sin that's carefully hidden that kills a person's soul more readily than the one that is aired for anyone to see.

When we begin to walk the spiritual path to managing our weight, we need to toss aside our secrets. God has little use for hypocrites—people who try to hide their secret sins. Often it is these same people who are so hard on other people's alleged sins. Jesus warned us about looking for specks in the eyes of others when we can't see the logs in our own eye. Or, in the case of weight loss, it would be like the person who criticizes others for having cream in their coffee when they, themselves, have just devoured three donuts that morning that no one was around to see.

Jesus didn't just criticize hypocrites because their behavior was driving a wedge between them and other people. Their secret behavior was also driving a wedge between them and God. To grow close to God, it is imperative that we become more and more open about who we are. The old saying that God can't drive a parked car applies equally well to the fact that God can't drive a car that has a tarp over it either. God knows your secrets, but you can't have a true relationship with Him when key events in your life are unspoken and hidden.

One of the most frightening challenges about the spiritual path to weight loss for some people is to give up their secrets. For such folks—perhaps you are one of them—hidden eating is what makes them feel like life is all right. They put their trust and faith in their hoard of cookies and chips. It's there for them when they have a fight with their husband or wife or are angry with their children. It comforts them if work went poorly that day or if some other disappointment came their way. Perhaps that is why trust is one of the first things that God demands we give to him. God wants us to trust Him instead of some crumpled bag of potato chips.

If you have stores of secret food, now's the time to clean house. Just open the drawer or cupboard or purse and take the food out, and toss it in the garbage can.

A PRAYER FOR THOSE WITH SECRET FOOD

One of my friends wrote the following prayer and used it to help her get through those times when she had to give up her secret food stores. I'd like to share it with you: "Lord, uncover the secrets of my heart. Know me as I am and let me know you as you are. Help me to rely on you instead of my chips and Kisses."

She taped that prayer to the cupboard door where she used to hide the bags of corn chips and chocolate Kisses that no one ever knew about (she told me she liked the chocolate Kisses and used to eat bags of them because they're so small they seemed hardly like anything). Habit would make her reach for that cupboard door when she was unhappy, and she'd see the prayer instead. She would stand right there and pray, asking God to help her trust Him to comfort her instead of the food she used in the past.

Don't try to convince yourself that instead of wasting the food you should eat it. If you truly can't stand to throw it out, give it to a friend or neighbor. Remember, I'm not going to suggest you throw out all the "good" stuff (read "bad" stuff) and then go on a diet. Besides, I hope that by now we're both in agreement about the disastrous effects of diets. You're simply getting your house in order as you take yet another step down your path to weight loss.

ELAINE'S STORY

*"So have no fear of them; for nothing is covered up
that will not be uncovered, and nothing secret that
will not become known.... Do not fear those who kill
the body but cannot kill the soul; rather fear him who
can destroy both soul and body in hell."*
Matthew 10:26, 28

When I think of the damage "secrets" can cause I am
reminded of a woman I'll call Elaine. Elaine's main
addiction was watching television for hours at a time—
particularly the daily soaps that provided her with a
confusing fantasy life to help her cope. In fact, she
crossed the line of fantasy, actually putting herself into
certain character roles so intensely that she lived her life
around the soap-opera schedule. She would not answer
the phone during a particularly sultry segment and not
answer the doorbell during the broadcast, even if it was
a friend or neighbor who'd come to call. If she had to
miss a program, she'd set the VCR on record and watch
the tape later that night. She devoured the soap summary magazines she saw in the supermarket and kept
stacks of past issues next to her ten years of unread
National Geographic stored in the garage. While televi-

sion was a secondary addiction—as strong an example of intimacy with a non-intimate object as you could imagine—she kept her first addiction—food—going full strength. A double whammy coupled with yet another addiction: secret spending.

"Dear, I gave you a $20 bill yesterday, but you have all these cash receipts from the ATM totaling $100. You're sure taking a lot of money out, aren't you?"

"Well, you know, honey, I had to buy an expensive present for Johnny's friend's birthday." (Actually spent $5.00—not mentioned.) "And then I had to get a full tank of gas." (Actually only spent $6.25—not mentioned.) "And then I paid cash for a costly dress for Susan." (Actually spent $9.50 at cut-rate store—not mentioned.) "You know, the charges really added up."

Elaine simply lied with half-truths. Yes, she bought some things. But they didn't cost as much as she implied. In fact, she bought cheap items all around, totaling only $20.75. The rest of the ATM money went for junk food that she quickly squirreled away under the bed, in the attic, in the garage, and even in the trunk of her car. While there was always a grain of truth in response to her husband's inquiries about money, Elaine's retort always seemed to be couched in a bigger, bolder lie—yet another co-addiction. Does any of this resonate with you?

For your emotional growth, and your ~~loss~~, it's important that you recognize y~~ou~~ up your secrets. They have interfered wit~~h~~ sabotaged your success. You have tried you~~r~~ what you thought would work, but nothing h~~as been~~ effective. In fact, your compulsive behavior has pro~~bab~~ly exacerbated the problem, not solved it. Now is the time to say, "I need help."

There's no need—and no point—to blame your past, your family, or even your former abuser, if any. You have simply had numerous unmet needs that you attempted to address with food. Now, you are moving away from such erroneous, ineffective thinking, and are moving toward the vulnerability and openness of honesty. You want more than anything to get out of your emotional tailspin and unhappy, cumulative years of flying recklessly on automatic pilot.

In 1994, the average American consumed almost 22 pounds of salt snacks (such as potato chips, popcorn, and pretzels)—a 4-pound increase from 1988. The most popular restaurant orders that same year were carbonated beverages, french fries, hamburgers, pizzas, and side salads. (Statistics from the U.S. Department of Agriculture)

For Elaine, it was necessary to engage in several high-dive experiences that challenged past beliefs with new,

encounters to help create a shift in her think-
behavior. We began our high dives wherever
was fear, hurt, misunderstanding, or frustration.
Elaine convinced herself that her problem was not
out weight but about her inability to let others really
see her, she became open to change and the weight just
began to drop off.

LOOKING BACK TO GO FORWARD

*"The world breaks everyone, and afterward
many are strong at the broken places."*
—*Ernest Hemingway*

We've already talked about how your past can trigger
compulsive behaviors related to food and other addictions. To the extent that your past programming has
torpedoed your life and caused you to hurt yourself by
acting out your pain by gravitating to food, I want to say
one important thing: In my experience, people with
obsessive-compulsive behaviors have suffered some
form of abuse. That's the past I want you to look at with
new eyes.

For you, the compulsion has become a love affair
with food. For others it may gambling, excessive risk-

taking, thrill-seeking, workaholism, chaotic living, or over-spending. Compulsive behaviors are actions that produce fairly intensive emotional arousal or emotional release. But it is not a healthy arousal. Compulsive behaviors always create anger, guilt, and long-term emotional pain. This is why a compulsive overeater may develop co-addictions as well, which means the gambling, excessive risk-taking, thrill-seeking, workaholism, chaotic living, and over-spending may be equally familiar to you.

Here's a key thought: All trauma causes us to seek relief. The question is how will you seek that relief? You and I do everything for one of two reasons: It is either *tension relieving* or *goal achieving.* If you release tension through food just because it feels good, is easy to do, and demands no thought on your part, then that decision will just make you fatter, unhappier, and more prone to blame others for your problems; it will continue to propel you toward personal failure and hopelessness.

If, however, you live your life with a sense of goal achieving, you then shift your focus to hope and a brighter, more confident future. That's why this prayer is so wonderful: "Lord, you give me the awareness to perceive and the strength to believe. I trust you completely to help me achieve."

In that same vein, what the slimy caterpillar calls doomsday is what we eventually see as an exquisite butterfly. We all get broken. At some time in our lives each of us slips into the dark cocoon of night, thinking we have little or no hope for a resurrection. But because we choose not to give up, we find there really is joy in the morning. What was ugly now becomes a thing of beauty. Where there was hate and disgust there is now hope and joy and the promise of a new tomorrow.

RECOVERY WILL KEEP YOU BUSY

If it is to be, it's up to me.

By now you may be saying, "It's starting to become clear. Food is not—nor has it ever been—my problem. It's something deeper, something I've not addressed, not admitted, not dealt with. Well, I'm now ready to make a move in the right direction. I want to start down that spiritual path to weight loss." If that is where you are in your thinking, then you are ready to work with the following checklist for recovery as you move from abusing food to freedom in asking God to help you deal with your addictions. I encourage you to begin to do the following:

- Learn to be free in expressing what you believe about yourself and the rigid set of rules you have chosen to live by up until now.

- Find a safe place—or safe person—to begin breaking your formal rules for survival. To hang on to the rules made by people who may no longer even be alive could be one of your greatest stressors. If it is a "father" or "mother" issue, you may want to talk to their portrait and tell them about your new direction. If they are deceased, you may need to write a letter to them and read it standing on or near their graves to get closure. Start breaking old, ineffective, untrue rules now.

- Expose yourself to people who believe in you and have your best interests at heart. These may be people in a social club, book study, or perhaps it is a special neighbor. Ask yourself if, say, Mary is safe for you. If she is, open yourself up to Mary little by little.

- Quit taking the blame for all the stuff that's gone on in your life. You are only one actor in a great stage play with many actors in elaborate costumes (which include masks) who speak both provocative and confounding dialogue. These people have come and gone across the stage during your entire life. You didn't write the play. You're not directing the play. In fact, you did not even ask to be in the play. So don't assume that you are responsible for the play. The only part in the production for which you are responsible is you, and that's how people who lose weight effectively view their presence on the stage of life.

People who lose weight effectively have come to live with hope. They don't deny the past; they deal with it. They make no rigid rules for present and future growth, they just grow.

If you continue to focus on the pain of your compulsive behaviors, you will make limited progress, if any, and your sense of loss, hopelessness, and fear will go on unabated. Compulsive overeaters are afraid they will never get out of their prisons of compulsive overeating.

What will you find as you look into your past? You may discover you've actually ritualized your eating behaviors. Overeating may have been your way to avoid anxiety, fear, and anger—all forms of addiction. What a sad, but nonetheless creative, way to hide your feelings! Up until now, you have shut out the emptiness in your life by your understandable fear of opening an emotional can of worms. It has been a form of body-numbing. You've turned off your body and your sexuality. You've done your best to make yourself nonsexual as you've reshaped yourself into someone whom no one could ever love again.

But now that you've made the commitment to go down the spiritual path to weight loss, you have decided it's OK to be you—to recognize your immense value and your big, caring heart. It's been my experience as a counselor that secret anger and resentment about the past is almost always a key issue that keeps a patient from going beyond the words of this chapter, and on to what could be great success in their emotional growth. You have now read 13 chapters in this book, which means you have demonstrated you have what it takes to start the spiritual path to weight loss. You dare to be brave. You dare to engage in yet one more high-dive experience. You dare to take adult responsibility for your actions, regardless of what may have happened to you as a child. And you are becoming secure enough in yourself to ask for help from a counselor, a friend, and from a God who made you and loves you.

Congratulations on your progress thus far. You have begun the spiritual path that will take you to a healthier lifestyle. That path will have some turns on it. We'll talk about that briefly in the next chapter and show how your comfort with your body is related to weight issues.

When Beauty Isn't Skin Deep

"The turn came for each girl to go in to King Ahasuerus, after being 12 months under the regulations for the women, since this was the regular period of their cosmetic treatment, six months with oil of myrrh and six months with perfumes and cosmetics for women."

Esther 2:12

YOUR POWER VERSUS STAR POWER

God made Cybill Shepherd to be Cybill Shepherd; God made you to be you.

*E*sther isn't alone in her quest for beauty. I recently saw a woman's magazine with a headline on the cover that promised, "Take off five pounds fast! Melt away your Thanksgiving binge." Inside was a full-color piece entitled, "Celebrity Inspiration: How the stars drop five pounds fast," a holiday feature found in the pages of *Woman's World*. For Shelley Fabares, it's a "magic drink" that keeps her at her ideal weight of 118 pounds. Candice Bergen turns to her "Paris plan," a bowl of onion soup for lunch and dinner and a banana or apple for breakfast. Dolly Parton likes to "juice it up" by enjoying squeezed orange juice for breakfast, papaya juice for lunch, and a glass of apple cider for dinner for up to five days to stay at her trim 105 pounds. A sub-head tells us that Whitney Houston likes to "binge on eggs," and when Sharon Stone wants to lose a quick five, she sits down to a sumptuous meal of celery and carrots.

These are the quick-fix, lose-five-pounds-fast regi-mens of just a few of the 12 ravishing women featured in the article, and at first glance, their methods of attacking fat may seem to be just the ticket for optimum weight management. Who wouldn't want a surefire way to lose a fast five pounds? It all seems so right, so OK, so all-American. However, what alarms me is one of the cap-tions over the full-color pictures of the ever-so-thin Dolly Parton, Joan Collins, Cybill Shepherd, and Sharon Stone that reads, "Lose that holiday weight and look great with diet strategies from the experts: stars who have to look slim for parties, parts, and public appearances."

Here's my concern. Marketing their images by appearing trim and sexy and latching on to various diets to guarantee their thinness are obviously important for the beautiful celebrity women who grace the pages of the magazine. But for the article to attempt to tie you to their overnight strategies so that you, too, will look good during the holidays—or any other day of the year—is deceptive. It is an attempt to span an almost unbridgeable gap. It may or may not work for you. If you do achieve overnight success with one of these plans, the diet could hook you inappropriately and catapult you into yet another backwash of dieting gimmicks. If it doesn't work—and the article makes no promise it will—then it's just one more fad you've tried and failed at. The piece talks nothing about looking "healthy" for the holidays but focuses only on the quickest way to lose five pounds.

Is this article going to ruin your life? I don't think so. Because some of the women also talk about how important exercise is for their complete regimen of weight management. However, if you read articles like this over and over, week after week, and try every diet that suggests overnight success so that you, too, can achieve and maintain your own personal celebrity look, then, yes, it will do you harm—especially if you are already challenged with obsessive-compulsive behavior.

The women in the three-page spread are beautiful. They are expensively coifed, gorgeously attired, slim, big-busted, and slender. What woman wouldn't like to have the shape of these Hollywood beauties?

But the people who lose weight successfully learn to turn the pages fast when they encounter these sirens of weight loss, beckoning the unprepared toward the rocks of dieting disaster. That's because people who lose weight successfully are no longer obsessed with their outer beauty, their waist size, how much they eat, when they eat it, dress measurements, bust size, what they must wear to cover fat, or how they must lose x inches of girth to be presentable at parties or feel good about themselves at public appearances.

> Do you find yourself envying the stars? Write down three things that you like about your own body. Especially things that you think you have that the stars don't. And keep the list around, perhaps in your journal, so that you can add to the list as you think of more things.

The pictures in the magazine are pretty, and the headlines are enticing, but the road to healthy—and sustainable—weight loss does not follow the paths of the stars.

THE STARS AND CHRISTIANS

Physical beauty withers and dies. Spiritual beauty lasts an eternity.

Why even mention this, you say? Don't Christians have enough sense not to be taken in by Hollywood's hype? Yes and no. Everyone likes to look attractive, and I believe God applauds us in that—after all, he made us attractive to look at! But when we become so intent on looking glamorous that we're willing to sacrifice even a little bit of our health, we need to re-think what we're doing.

The average person coming to me for counseling for weight challenges has been on at least seven diets. These men and women have learned to count calories automatically, have an obsession with cholesterol, know as much about packaged diet foods as the manufacturers of those foods, have fasted, eaten only herbs, wracked their bodies with faddish liposuction, and have had their stomachs stapled. Desperate people do desperate things. The trouble is that most desperate people do the wrong things. People who lose weight effectively get off the roller-coaster diet ride. People who lose weight and keep it off realize their lives must no longer revolve around food.

People who start down the spiritual path to weight loss know they must take control of their lives and start living as God, their heavenly Father and faithful Friend, intends them to live, with freedom, joy, and an all abiding sense of self-worth.

People who go down that path recognize the deceit of diets and no longer choose to be victimized by one of the most unregulated industries on record. We now know that women who watch TV ads about dieting or diet products eat nearly twice as much as those who watch ads about other consumer products. Your first line of defense if you are one of these victims? Change the channel. It can be your first step toward taking control of your new life.

An obsession with dieting has never worked, and it never will. Diets hurt you mentally and physically. You lose the weight; you gain it back. You feel good about yourself for a moment, and then you feel terrible. Diets are a cruel joke of bait and switch. You've been conned into thinking you are buying one thing and end up stuck with something else. Have you ever thought of this? If diets worked, everyone would be thin. Diets are a kind of Russian roulette.

And the game can be deadly. Yet, somehow we figure the odds are in our favor so we pay our money and take our chances. We're seduced by full-page, full-color promises, paid celebrity testimonials, newspaper and glamour magazine advertisements, and European "miracle" stories of instant fat removal. There is no end to the deceit. Nor is there a lack of the vulnerable who'll do anything to be thin and therefore be loved, admired, and accepted.

People who lose weight and keep it off have quit grazing in the diet aisle of their local bookstore. They turn the page fast when they come across a diet ad in a magazine. They change the channel immediately when a paid celebrity spokesperson speaks of the miraculous results of the latest, greatest, most foolproof weight loss program in history.

People who are on the spiritual path to weight loss learn to become more decisive, more selective, more in tune with themselves. They decide to face their most frantic fears because they know it is the only way they will ever address their deepest pain.

They look their shame, jealousy, rage, and anger in the eye and call it for what it is. Why do they do this? Because they now know their internal angst has compelled them to think less than kindly of themselves and has forced them to turn to food as their friend.

Whether you're 20 or 200 pounds overweight—and you don't like what you see in the mirror—it's OK not to be proud of your temporary appearance. That's because now you are learning that the outward manifestation of who you are for the moment does not reflect the kind, loving, good-hearted person you are inside. The good news is that you can change your outward appearance, and you are already on that path to weight loss, because you are now focusing on health not fads, on being a model for yourself and not worshiping the magazine models who do not have your best interest at heart. You now know that comparing yourself to anyone or anything is a fast track to misery, and you do not choose to be miserable any longer.

MARSHA'S STORY

Just because the concept is simple, doesn't necessarily mean it's easy.

Having made this decision to avoid comparing yourself with others, you are immediately less vulnerable to the thin-equals-sexy land mines that have been planted across the vast advertising and promotional landscape just waiting to explode in your face one more time. It is also a decision you will need to make day after day because successful weight loss is a journey of a lifetime and not a day trip.

People who succeed in losing weight know the concept is simple, but not necessarily easy, because those land mines of deceit, funded by a money-crazed Madison Avenue, will forever be laid at their feet. That's why people who lose weight and keep it off don't go it alone. They read books like this one that provide real promise and real hope. They seek and listen to counseling that focuses on the whole person. They throw away the diet books. They learn to read the labels in the supermarket. They don't watch diet ads on television. Instead of nibbling endlessly on high-calorie, high-fat snack foods, they eat carrots, sticks of celery, raisins, fruit, and other nutritious foods from God's bountiful creation. Why? Because they have learned to like their bodies and know that their present condition is only temporary. They have learned the art of self-acceptance. They compare themselves with no one. No one!

I wish Marsha (not her real name) had learned not to compare herself with others earlier. Here is a summary of what she told me in a private session. I share these thoughts with you with her permission.

> EVERY TIME I WENT *to the supermarket, I would buy a copy of the latest tabloid and at least two or three glamour or fitness magazines. Because I had a weight problem I*

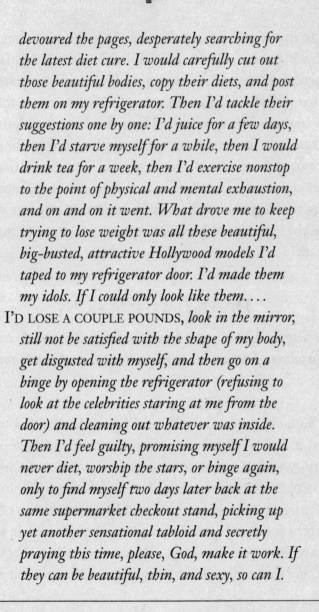

devoured the pages, desperately searching for the latest diet cure. I would carefully cut out those beautiful bodies, copy their diets, and post them on my refrigerator. Then I'd tackle their suggestions one by one: I'd juice for a few days, then I'd starve myself for a while, then I would drink tea for a week, then I'd exercise nonstop to the point of physical and mental exhaustion, and on and on it went. What drove me to keep trying to lose weight was all these beautiful, big-busted, attractive Hollywood models I'd taped to my refrigerator door. I'd made them my idols. If I could only look like them....

I'D LOSE A COUPLE POUNDS, *look in the mirror, still not be satisfied with the shape of my body, get disgusted with myself, and then go on a binge by opening the refrigerator (refusing to look at the celebrities staring at me from the door) and cleaning out whatever was inside. Then I'd feel guilty, promising myself I would never diet, worship the stars, or binge again, only to find myself two days later back at the same supermarket checkout stand, picking up yet another sensational tabloid and secretly praying this time, please, God, make it work. If they can be beautiful, thin, and sexy, so can I.*

In my years of counseling I have had the privilege of working with some remarkable people who've faced unspeakable adversity and painful memories to come to grips with their life in the present. Many were so intent on looking like those thin, sexy vixens in the glamour magazines that they started to walk a path leading to personal destruction. For many, their eating disorders had already become full-blown anorexia or bulimia. It was no longer simply an obsessive compulsion with weight or overeating; it had become a matter of life and death.

DEALING WITH SUCCESS

Losing weight is not an end in itself; it's merely a by-product of other, more important transformations.

Suppose you've lost 10 or 20 pounds. You are trim, you're feeling great, you walk with more spring in your step, you feel more confident than ever, and then—wham! A handsome co-worker—who never paid much attention to you before—now detains you at the office water cooler and begins to express some interest in you. Scary, for you, perhaps. When you were carrying around those extra pounds you did not have to deal with the attention. In fact, you may have put on weight in the past for that purpose. Now what do you do? Run? Seek cover? Or will you learn to trust yourself with your weight loss. This is a very important issue for you to prepare for because you may feel as if you have a new body and not know how to respond to the attention. In fact you do have a new body. You are going through a significant transformation.

What happens if you lose weight and your spouse suddenly begins treating you differently—good or bad? What are your greatest fears? What happens if you become so attractive you are literally scared to death? It's possible that your fears may suddenly become quite high, and as your fear goes up so may your weight. That's often how it works. But it doesn't have to be that way. That's why there are at least three critical levels of fortification that must occur for you along the way:

> Discontent makes rich men poor, while contentment makes poor men rich. Don't let fear and intimidation separate you from the riches of your own contentment.

• Don't lose weight in anger. It will short-circuit your progress. If someone says to you, "Gee, you're looking nice. Have you lost weight?" It's easy for you to hear those words as a put down. Instead, reframe them. Say to yourself, "If he only knew what was really going on. Yes, I've lost weight, but that's only a by-product of other—more important—things I'm dealing with." Remind yourself that you're now dealing with your success, not living with former failure.

• Say goodbye to resentment. As you begin to lose weight, the intensity of your emotions may increase to the level where you may feel you are even more out of control than in the past. Further, you'll need to remember that you have no control over how others will respond to you as you lose weight. Some will be rude: "Lost your double chin, eh?" "What's the matter, no more french fries and malts?" "Wow, you must have really had a weight problem, because you look so good now." Remember, some people will not know what to say to you. So you'll need to learn to take care of yourself while caring for others. It's not going to be easy, but it is the attitude of people who lose weight successfully.

• Don't live the hermit's life. Your previous weight problem may have been simply an outward manifestation of other emotional challenges that you are now dealing with from a fresh, new perspective. You've made great progress, so stay with the program. You want the opposite of a hermit's life. You're working for an integration of the total you: body, soul, and spirit. You need to join in, not separate yourself.

As you learn to deal successfully and effectively with your success, your self-esteem will rise and your self-confidence will carry you on. It will not necessarily be easy, but the reward will be a thousand times greater than the effort.

Part of the spiritual path to weight loss is to face our fears, especially the ones that are difficult for us. If it is your goal to be a person who's committed to emotional growth—which is the beginning of the spiritual path of weight loss—for the rest of your life, this could indeed be difficult for you. But it is a risk you must take if you choose to come to grips with the real issues at stake.

ONE STEP AT A TIME

All shadows of doubt can be replaced by the light of your growing personal confidence as you remain true to who and what you are becoming.

You can start out small. Let's say you're threatened by people who are especially good-looking. If that's the case, make a conscious attempt to attend a social gathering at church, at the office, or in the community where these people will be present. You don't even have to talk to them. Just be in the social setting as a relaxed, comfortable person who deserves to be there without being intimidated. Remember, what you fear about the other person probably has nothing to do with his or her feelings toward you. Practice being the loving, open-hearted person you are becoming. Recognize your boundaries, and do not let the other person take from you emotionally.

Sometimes it's not the fear of being noticed that troubles people. Sometimes it's the fear that you can't trust yourself. "If I begin to lose weight and actually begin enjoying the attention I receive from the opposite sex am I compromising my values? How do I know I won't succumb to a subtle manipulation from others?" There is no need to compromise your values if, with God's help, you remain committed to your goal of effective weight loss and personal spiritual growth. This will, however, be one of those high-dive experiences that you'll have to go through. You will learn a lot about yourself, and yes, it may be frightening at first. But just because you lose weight, your values do not need to change. Up until now you have been hiding your God-given sexuality behind a wall of fat. Now you have the exciting privilege of being—and expressing—the whole person you've always been.

This is emotional health of the highest order, and now, perhaps for the first time, you are starting to walk this exciting, new spiritual path to weight loss. Congratulations on your decision, because the best is yet to come. As I will mention in the next chapter, the spiritual path to weight loss is lined with increased happiness. Read it with me—with joy and hope—and you'll see what I mean.

On That Day God Made Chocolate—And It Was Good

"It is good to give thanks to the Lord, and to sing praises to your name, O Most High."

Psalm 92:1

BREATHE DEEPLY

It's hard to jump for joy when your body doesn't feel like jumping at all.

A young woman, I'll call her Mary, sat in my office chair one day and said to me, "I wish I were dead." Instead of responding immediately to her feelings, I asked her if it would be all right if I turned on some music. I found an upbeat radio station that was playing a song with a strong rhythm. Then I asked Mary if she'd do me a favor. Intrigued by now, she agreed. I asked her to start doing some mild aerobic exercises with me. After a couple of minutes, I stopped both of us.

"Can you feel that?" I asked.

"What?" she answered back.

"Take a breath," I replied and we both breathed deeply. "Your heart. Your muscles. They love being alive! Your body loves being alive!"

Of course, that wasn't the end of the conversation with Mary, only the beginning. A few weeks later, Mary came into my office all excited. She'd driven out to a forest area, sat down, and breathed in the smell of the pine trees. Another day she stood outside in the rain and felt the rain falling on her face. On still another day, she'd dug in the dirt and discovered earthworms. Within a short period of time, Mary found she'd begun to celebrate life.

I can almost see you scratching your head now, saying, "But Dr. Jantz, what's that got to do with me? I'm not suicidal. I'm not wishing I were dead. All I want to do is lose some weight."

The reason I'm telling you about Mary is that, in my experience, many people who are overweight have pushed back the senses that put them in touch with life. Extra weight can serve as a cocoon wrapped around you to protect yourself. But those layers of fat might also be separating you from some of the physical joys of life—

like the joy of feeling your heart pump after exercise or feeling your muscles work hard, or the simple pleasure of taking a walk through the woods or a stroll on the beach. In short, your extra weight may be dampening your natural enthusiasm to celebrate life.

THE HALLELUJAH CHORUS AND YOU
As sure as God puts His children into the furnace of affliction, He will be with them there.

One of the tests of knowing whether someone is on the spiritual path to weight loss or not is to listen for an increase in laughter and in positive, emotionally healthy, life-giving, joyous statements. The closer we draw to God, the closer we draw to pure, unfiltered joy. When you're on that path, you just may find yourself humming the Hallelujah chorus without even thinking about it.

> God is before me,
> He will be my guide;
> God is behind me,
> no ill can betide;
> God is beside me,
> to comfort and cheer;
> God is around me,
> so why should I fear?

Let me emphasize the underlying joy we have with God as our guide. This joy does not mean that you will be without problems. More often than not, weight issues are tied to other concerns in your life, and when you begin to lose weight (or even think about losing weight) many of these once-dormant issues may begin to surface. It's been my observation, though, that even with that sadness or grief, there is a growing bedrock of joy in a person who sets out on the spiritual journey to weight loss. God is more than our guide; He is our reason for thanksgiving.

This thanksgiving does not come instantaneously. In fact, you may not even recognize it as thanksgiving at first. The process of uncovering the thankful person inside you reminds me of a story I read once:

It seems there was an artist who one day found that a large piece of granite had risen unexpectedly from the yard outside his home. Now, I don't know about you, but if that had happened to me I'd be upset. Just one more annoying thing I'd need to take care of before I could mow the lawn. Reportedly, it did annoy the artist, and he knew he'd eventually have to do something about it. He debated about borrowing a jackhammer from a friend until he remembered that, of course, he had no friends with jackhammers. Then he thought about getting some dynamite and blasting the granite into smaller stones that he could then carry away. But that didn't seem right either so he sat and thought about what to do. As he sat and thought and looked at that stone, he began to look past his problem. He forgot about his goal of getting rid of the stone. He actually started to see the stone. He noticed the lines and the shape. He decided the stone wasn't so bad after all. He decided to be grateful for the stone. Then one day he got out his chisel and hammer, and within a short time, he created an unbelievable reproduction of an elephant. Neighbors and passersby alike were amazed when they saw what appeared to be a real elephant grazing in his yard.

A friend asked the amateur sculptor how he'd managed to do such a good job in reproducing a realistic form of an elephant without even a model or picture to go by. The artist replied confidently, "It was really pretty easy, actually. I just chipped away everything that didn't look like an elephant."

Got any elephants in there? I like this story because it illustrates what we've been saying in all our previous chapters. Right now, there are still rocks, barriers, walls, and other impediments in your life that keep hanging you up, keeping you from reaching your life's goals, and thwarting you from losing weight. These are things and events you can't seem to get around, go over, crawl under, or tunnel through. Yet, they are not obstacles to be done away with. Instead, they need to be creatively handled, just as the sculptor was creative in cutting away what didn't look like an elephant. So my question to you is, What elephants do you have waiting to emerge from what now appears to be just a chunk of annoying rock? Or, if you don't like elephants, what flower, healthy relationship, or big, loving heart is waiting to come from what you may have seen as a nuisance until now?

We all need to take inventory of our lives and sculpt away that which is threatening and hurtful to us to get closer to what is important, productive, and growth-producing for our lives. It's those parts of our lives for which we can be thankful. Here's the key thought for this chapter: If you are serious about continuing your walk on this spiritual path to weight loss, you will work hard to chip away everything that does not look like the person you most wish to become. As you do this, you are saying goodbye to the kind of thinking that may have already given you high blood pressure or heart disease, or is about to do so.

In the past, you may not have been aware of the close correlation between your body and soul. But now you have a new insight. You know that if you are to enjoy weight-loss success in the long term, you will be aware that God has made you a complicated, intricate, unique human being where there is virtually no boundary between body and soul. You are you, and there are no divisions, mental or physical. This means you have given up the game of "getting even" with those who would do you harm. Not even President Lincoln could hold a grudge, it seems, for he even put his political enemies, Stanton, Chase, and Seward, into his presidential cabinet.

Disraeli, the brilliant English prime minister, went out of his way to do favors for those who bitterly opposed him. When once asked how he dealt with his most intractable foes, the British statesman said, "I never trouble to be avenged. When a man injures me, I put his name on a slip of paper and lock it up in a drawer. It is marvelous to see how the men I have so labeled have a way of disappearing."

BELIEVE IT IN YOUR BONES

"For as he thinketh in his heart, so is he."
Proverbs 23:7 (KJV)

The good news is that you, too, can make this transformation, because people much like you have already done it or are in the process of turning their lives around. You are not alone—you are not the first one in this experiment—even though we are talking about a new type of life for many of you.

Healthy, growing people who lose weight successfully no longer wallow in past trauma—no matter how terrible it was. They allow the pain to heal so they can put it to rest and get on with their lives. They ultimately come to the point where they de-label themselves. No longer are they "compulsive," "obsessive," or afflicted with an "eating disorder." This is not denial. It's emotional health, and a determination to begin living life in the present. Diets and gadgets will never help you achieve your goal of effective weight loss. But your commitment to whole-person thinking—and subsequent follow-through action—will.

When you decide to believe in your bones that healthy people are growing people, you'll have a more positive, realistic view of yourself. You may still feel shy and self-conscious at first, but if you keep moving forward, you will be able to see your pain and call it for what it is. As you move forward, you'll also discover that a new, healthy excitement will come your way as you begin to maintain more appropriate boundaries. Part of your maturing process will come when you know on which lines to fight the battle.

Science and psychology both remind us that the brain cannot make a clear distinction between an established fact and a dominant desire. Therefore, as you verbally give thanks, you are telling your brain that you are a thankful person who is losing weight and enjoying God's gifts. You see yourself as a successful person. In your mind's eye you have already arrived at your desired goal.

Unless you already see yourself as complete, whole, loving, joyous, and lovable now, your goal of weight loss will be forever elusive. The saying Rome wasn't built in a day is rendered into Chinese as an overweight person did not get there with one bite. Same message. It takes time to gain, and it takes time to lose. But time is on your side.

Besides, being thin does not guarantee you'll be satisfied with your body shape or your life, nor does being a few pounds over suggest that you have a poor self-concept. What seems to be of greatest significance, according to several recent studies, is how much your parents, relatives, and those closest to you emphasized your appearance as a child—how you were conditioned to think about your looks.

Now, as one who is on your way to effective weight loss, you know the past is past and the present is the present. Whatever was done is done; whatever was said was said. The sooner you quit focusing on your body—or what ancient history may have said about it—the sooner you'll make quality time available for important things in your life.

REBECCA'S STORY

Are you committed to cutting away those things that, up until now, have prohibited you from losing weight?

One of my patients, Rebecca, wrote in her journal the following sequence of thoughts of how one day the light went on as she started looking at her life. With her permission, I share her thoughts with you:

> DR. JANTZ POINTED OUT *to me that my self-worth at one time was based entirely on what I looked like. If I was thin and attractive, I felt acceptance from myself and others. It seemed so much easier to focus on my appearance, on my outside. My insides were so out of kilter anyway that I couldn't even think about them. If I focused on my body, my weight, food, purging, and exercising, then I didn't have to think about what was wrong with me.*
> I DIDN'T UNDERSTAND *what was happening to me because the pain was so hard to face. It wasn't until I was in a safe place, with people I felt secure with and who knew how to help me,*

> *that I could unlock that pain, take a look at it, and reveal the truth.*
>
> UNDERSTANDING THE REASONS *for my behavior has helped me to deal with the guilt I felt all those lost years. It has helped me to deal with the guilt I felt over being a "bad" little girl, with the fear that people won't accept me unless I'm thin. When I finally realized how anger, fear, and guilt contributed to my eating disorder and how my eating disorder had numbed my anger, I was finally able to get off that endless merry-go-round of eating disorders. But it not only helped me. I also began to understand the weight challenges of my ten-year-old daughter. For that insight alone, I thank God.*

I shared with Rebecca something I'm going to share with you now. These are four principles for losing weight:

• People who start down the spiritual path to weight loss have learned they do not need to—nor can they—fix everything now or ever. They have become realistic about their own assets and liabilities. This is the first step to inner peace.

• People who start down this path also agree that their lives have simply not been working well at all.

Their lifestyle has been killing them physically and emotionally, deadening their sensibilities to themselves and others. They've learned to stop long enough to feel real pain so they could deal with it.

• People who walk the spiritual path to effective weight loss learn to respect and accept themselves as unique creations of a loving heavenly Father. They see themselves as recipients of some of God's greatest gifts. They are grateful for what's wonderful about them and are ready to improve on what is not. The most dramatic result arising from this new awareness is that their lives begin to change. Joy becomes a new word in their vocabulary, followed by peace, contentment, and rest.

• People who walk the spiritual path to weight loss admit their lives have not been manageable, and that they need help. They've coped for years with diets, exercise equipment, advertising hype, and trying to model the models, but it was an exercise in futility. They just gained more weight. The truth, however, is those things were always worse than they'd imagined. When they finally confronted the pain face to face, happiness and personal fulfillment were standing close by to greet them with open arms.

Earlier in this chapter, I told you the story of the amateur sculptor who chiseled an elephant out of granite. You'll remember that when asked how he did it, he said, "It was really pretty easy, actually. I just chipped away everything that didn't look like an elephant." What have you started to chip away at as you've read this chapter? What do you see emerging? Do you like what is appearing? Are you committed to cutting away those things that up until now have prohibited you from losing weight? Perhaps you will discover some of the answers in the next chapter as you write the story of your journey thus far.

That's the Story of Your Life

*"The Lord hath called me before I was born, while I
was in my mother's womb he named me."*

Isaiah 49:1

WHO ARE YOU?

**"I had given diets too much power, scales too much
power, other people's opinions of me too much power,
calorie-counting too much power."**
—Linda

We define ourselves by many things in our lives:
our jobs, our relationships, our talents, our pos-
sessions.... And yet none of these things answers the
critical question, Who am I?

When you walk the spiritual path to weight loss, you
will find an increasing desire to know yourself better.
I'm not talking about becoming self-absorbed or nar-

cissistic. I am speaking of the kind of deep and honest self-knowledge that can free you to be the person God created you to be.

Throughout this book, I've shared several stories with you. Most people who set out on this spiritual path to weight loss end up writing their own stories, often as a means to understanding the issues and patterns that develop in their lives. I always suggest to people that they begin the story of their lives where their real lives actually began—with their parents and their childhood family. I am going to share one story, about a woman I'll call Linda, and then later, I'm going to help you write your own story.

> MY NAME IS LINDA, *and this is my story. I don't know how different it is from other stories you've heard, but it's the only one I have, and I've asked Dr. Jantz if I could share it with you. If I had told you two years ago about my 13 diets, the more than 100 bottles of diet pills I'd consumed, my constant binging, and the way I hid food in the garage, closets, and the attic, I would have spoken to you as a woman without hope. I'd tried everything under the sun to lose weight, and nothing worked. Absolutely nothing.*

FOUR YEARS AGO *I was 32 years old and was 85 pounds overweight. At one point I weighed 253 pounds. I was a very large woman. Whenever I'd look at my high school yearbook and see a picture of the slim 103-pound Linda, I would cry, truly believing I would never be thin again. I was convinced there was no hope for me. I hated myself and everything about me. My marriage was in ruins, my children didn't want to be seen in the same zip code with me, and my friends—the few I had— were becoming fewer every day.*

IF I HADN'T BEEN SUCH A COWARD, *I might have ended it all. But deep down there was a faint spark of hope that there might be something I had not yet tried that would be the key to unlock the prison door that kept me in bondage. I discovered the key to be something I'd never considered in my entire life: the thing I call the "control button" to my life.*

IT'S ALMOST WITH TEARS *I tell you this, because I got in touch with something deep inside. As I answered some of Dr. Jantz's questions about my childhood, I discovered that making decisions was a big area of concern for me. As a child, my parents had controlled my*

every move: what I wore, what I said, my
friends—the list is endless. I felt I was supposed
to be perfect at everything! As incredible as it
sounds, for the first time in memory, I was
making my own decisions about my life—small
as those decisions were: eating a healthy breakfast, not weighing myself, and choosing my
own activity for as long as I wanted to do it.

I STARTED TO FEEL GOOD about myself. Hey,
Linda, you're not so bad after all. Yes, you're
still fat, but something's happening to you
that's never happened before. You're taking
control of your life in a wonderful new way.
You've got the control button now.

I WOULD GO TO SEE DR. JANTZ once a week.
It was a great experience for me because I'd talk
about how relaxed I was starting to feel, how I
wasn't yelling at the kids as much, and even
though I still had challenges with my marriage
I had begun to enjoy a greater sense of well-
being. The funny thing was that Dr. Jantz and
I seldom talked about food. A weight-loss professional not talking about food? It was uncanny.
We talked instead about me, Linda—who I
was, who I was as a child, who I was as a wife,
who I am in my secret moments.

AFTER FOUR WEEKS *I realized I was starting to lose weight. Unbelievable. I had stopped "grazing" on food by nearly 50 percent and had become much less compulsive in my eating. I was no longer using a scale at all (it's still in Dr. Jantz's office, along with the scales of a dozen other of his clients, I believe). I realized for the first time what a judgmental device a scale actually is; always telling me whether I'm good or bad, up or down, this way or that. I was no longer into good or bad. I no longer aimed for perfection. My focus was how to take control of my life. I had given diets too much power, scales too much power, other people's opinions of me too much power, calorie-counting too much power. Now, I was moving toward progress with less and less thought of perfection.*

TO MAKE A LONG STORY SHORT, *after two years I had shed over 85 pounds and I've never felt or looked better in my life. I eat healthy foods, drink lots of water, exercise regularly, and no longer blame anyone for anything. Best of all, I now care about myself.*

SPOTLIGHT ON YOU

The spiritual path leads you through your troubles,
but it always comes out on the other side.

If you identified with parts of Linda's story, it's time to discover your own story (and we each have one). The following are some of the exercises that will help you discover the unique journey that is your life. Here's what I encourage you to do now to take full advantage of the experiences you've had along the journey:

• Divide your life into ten-year periods: Look for episodes of resentment (anger), fear, and guilt; any character traits (addictions or secrets) that could be tied to your unhappiness. Be completely honest with yourself and avoid self-deception. Make notes of your assets and your liabilities. Write out at least seven things you like very much about your personality in each period.

• Choose an appropriate listener—a trustworthy, non-family member who will keep what you share in confidence. Look for someone who will bring wisdom and hope while listening to you. Tell him or her your story. Acknowledge to the listener any fear, embarrassment, guilt, or whatever you may be feeling, and just begin. Start with childhood and work up to the present, remembering the purpose of this encounter is to allow for your healing, not to please or impress the listener.

• Decide to turn any addictive aspects of your personality into positive energy. Move toward people not toward food. What three people are you willing to turn to today? Make your list, along with specific ideas you want to communicate to them, now.

Over the years, I have developed a series of special exercises to help people look at their lives as children. The foundation of our lives are laid when we are children, and these years as so critical that I give them special emphasis when I talk with people. Following are some exercises that focus on your childhood:

Imagine that your parents are very old and do not have long to live. (Even if they are deceased, I encourage you to do this exercise anyway.) They are making a surprise visit to your home. Write out in detail what they might say to you. Touch those areas that have hurt you most. Here are five positive things that may happen to you during this exercise:

• You can give yourself permission to resume the position of executive director of your life.

• You can learn to forgive—whether your parents are alive or dead.

• You can free yourself from past hurts because you are finally writing the forgiveness script.

- You can release the poisons and toxins of the past and replace them with the power and strength of your newfound freedom.

- You can become aware that you no longer need to carry the burdens of the past, because you are free at last. The truth has set you free.

You will soon discover that just by looking with adult eyes at your past, you will uncover some amazing things. Take some time and write your answers to the following questions:

- How did your family's living patterns affect you? How are you still living out those patterns? Are you doing it unconsciously? Consciously?

- Write about your mother. Who was she? What were her strengths? Weaknesses? Have you made a healthy, grown-up separation from your mother? Or have you spent your life trying to make your mother happy? Do you still try to do this? Write out some examples. Does your mother create guilt for you today? If so, how does she do that? What's your response to that guilt? Do you respond with compulsive behaviors?

- Do you tell your mother when you disagree with her? Do you feel like your mother listened to you as a child? Does she listen to you today? If not, why do you think that is? Does she affirm you as you live your life today?

• How does your father make you feel physically? Is it a healthy response? Do you numb the feeling? Feel upset? Do you get sick to your stomach? Are you prone to headaches?

• How are your mother's expectations of you still affecting your life today? List three of your mother's favorite sayings that have had a negative effect on you? Write out three sayings that have had a positive effect.

• Which of your father's traits do you think you have?

• What did you learn about the spiritual side of life as you grew up? Did your family hold strict religious beliefs? What were they? Did they use certain labels to identify people? Denominational labels? Agnostic, atheistic labels? Was there a deep passion behind their religious thinking? Were they judgmental? Conservative? Liberal? Loving? Kind? Were your parents' religious beliefs consistent with their behavior?

What was this exercise like for you? Did it provide any new insights into your present behavior? For the overeater, unpleasant or incongruent childhood experiences are often the triggers that continue to drive them to food for solace and comfort as adults. For example, if your mother was highly critical of you, of your weight, and of all the ice cream you ate, then as an adult you may continue to go to that ice cream in anger, consciously or unconsciously. In fact, you may be so hooked into this past experience that even something as innocent as a phone conversation with your mother may trigger your urge to run to the fridge and eat a half-gallon of ice cream. That is the power of an unresolved past.

The good news in all of this is that the spiritual path to weight loss is a path that doesn't stop with your unhappy childhood. It's a path that walks through those troubles and comes out on the other side. God can help you walk past the pain of your childhood and stand as an adult now able to take control of your own life.

• Write out five ways in which you are different—in a positive way—from your parents or those who raised you. Be as specific as possible.

1. _____

2. _____

3. _____

4. _____

5. _____

• Write a letter of "freedom" to your parents, but do not give it to them unless you are working together with a counselor. Acknowledge that they did what they could, and much of it was good. However, there were also issues that were hurtful and damaging to you. Acknowledge this in a spirit of love. Talk about your newfound freedom from the negative events of the past, and how they no longer are allowed to be the fuel for your food addictions. Write how you have been liberated to become your own parent and are now ready to perform all requisite responsibilities that that role demands.

• Read this letter to a trusted friend. Then, together, go out to a safe place, such as a fishing pier, the seashore, on or the edge of a lake, and burn the letter. In front of your friend and witness say, I'm now letting go of my past and will no longer allow past hurt or abuse to direct my life. I am finally free to be the person God created me to be.

• After you've completed this action plan, give yourself a nonfood reward, such as going to a movie or a play, taking a long walk on the beach, or sharing some of your new insights with a friend. Whatever you do, take action, and do it in a spirit of joy and celebration.

When you say, "I care about myself. I am becoming the person I was meant to be. I like what God has created. I am a person who is on the spiritual path to weight loss," then a wonderful world of self-acceptance begins to unfold and carry you one step closer to your goal. The Book of Proverbs reminds us that as a person thinks in his heart, so is he. That's a very old saying, but no less true today than when it was written. Think good thoughts of yourself. Never put yourself down. What you think, you are. Your subconscious hears all and believes all. Treat it with respect. It is one of the most important parts of something called *you*.

As you continue to take one step at a time down this exciting spiritual path to effective weight loss, you'll discover a desire to make more friends, and an eagerness to spend more time with old ones. We are people who need people—no matter who we are. That's why the Church—the body of Christ—is so important for our individual growth. Ideally, the Church community is a place where you will find the kind of acceptance that re-enforces what you're learning about yourself as you walk your own unique spiritual path to permanent weight loss. In the next few chapters, we're going to spend some time thinking about the Church, and how we can help make it a place of love and acceptance for ourselves and others.

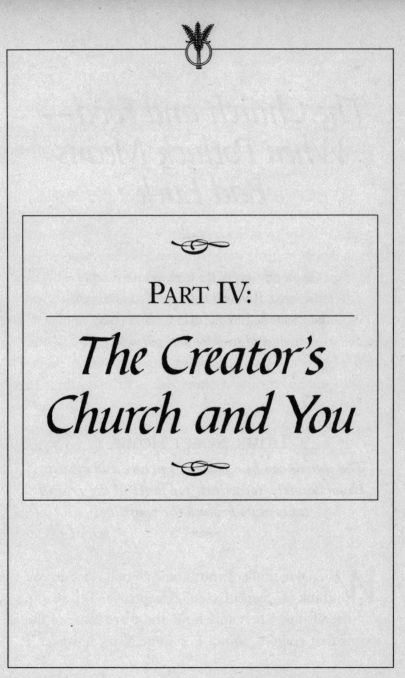

PART IV:

The Creator's Church and You

The Church and Food— When Potluck Means Bad Luck

"On the first day of the week, when we met to break bread, Paul was holding a discussion with them; since he intended to leave the next day, he continued speaking until midnight."

Acts 20:7

HOME, SWEET HOME

The church can be a place of nurture and growth. Unfortunately, sometimes too much of the growth takes place around the waistline.

When you think of your home church what do you think of? Sweet haven? Acceptance? Fellowship and friendship? I certainly hope those are some of the words that come to mind. For some of us, however, I fear, the words we think of may be disapproval, cliques, loneliness, and awkwardness.

For a person starting down the spiritual path to weight loss, there is no more important group of people than friends and colleagues in the local church. Don't ask me why God arranged it like this, but He made us people who need other people. The church, in its finest glory, is one of God's greatest gifts to us. It can be a place of true nurture and growth. Unfortunately, sometimes too much of the growth takes place around the waistline.

For many of us, the church offers temptations in the form of food. You may have thought, well, it's my church. Even in the earliest record of the church, fellowship included bread. Eating together has become a symbol of our community. So, when we go to church, we tend to think that we're supposed to have a great time there of fellowship, which includes nourishment both for the spirit as well as for the body.

It is a place for coming together with our spiritual concerns, so why not also enjoy it all—including the extra fellowship around the table? Unfortunately, though, that table has expanded over the years. It's no longer a Spartan table of bread and wine. Now, more often than not, the church table is loaded with chocolate donuts, angel food cake, apple pies, fried chicken dinners with mashed potatoes and gravy, salads heaped with mayonnaise, topped off with more ice cream than a fellowship-hungry person ought to have!

I have counseled many clients over the years who've told me that this scenario was their life: music and meringue, faith and fellowship, piety and pie! But before long, the fellowship of the overcomers becomes the fellowship of the overeaters. But they—and, perhaps you—always saw it as the social thing to do.

Then, one day, someone at church said, "Sister, you're putting on a few pounds, aren't you?" He may even have been blunt and said, "You know, I hate to say it, but you're getting fat!" Ouch! That hurt. It also confused you. You were doing what you thought was right:

THE OBLIGATION TO EAT

You've probably felt it before—in your church, at a social service club, or in your home. You heard someone say, "Honey, clean your plate. Don't you know there are millions of starving children in Africa who would just love to have that last morsel?" You may have taken the guilt to heart, which is then only a short distance down to your stomach. Is it possible that you have never left a plate empty since? Hunger is a valid reason to eat; guilt is not.

eating at church. If you were going to sin, you certainly wouldn't have done it in a place of worship. Your alleged "sin" was now out in the open, and you felt you were in good company. But the unkind comment started to make you feel some shame. Strangely, instead of moving away from food, you actually edged closer to it. In fact, that pattern may still be hurting you today.

ROLE MODELS—THIN-WAISTED DREAMS

Each person, regardless of his or her weight, has a special, often moving, story worth discovering and listening to.

Here's an exercise I want you to complete right now—while you are reading this page. This is for your eyes only, so please be honest with your response. List your five most likely role models, those people who you would like to be like physically:

_____

_____

_____

_____

_____

Who are your role models based on their physical appearance? Calcutta's late Mother Teresa? Israel's former Prime Minister Golda Meir? I don't think so. But if I suggested that they might be people such as Raquel Welch, Richard Gere, Jane Fonda, Tom Cruise—any of the tanned, toned, and thin stars in the Hollywood scene, I'd probably be getting closer to the kind of person you would most like to look like.

Of course, we'd all be quick to add that we don't want to be like them spiritually, or perhaps we wouldn't want to have their personality. But their bodies? Yes! We'd much rather have the body of a movie star than the body of a priest. Why? We simply don't expect godly people to be physically attractive. I'm going to repeat that because it is such a prevalent part of our Christian culture. *We somehow don't expect godly people to appear physically attractive.* Why? Because we're so used to seeing a split between that which is physical and that which is spiritual.

The reality is that the body of Christ, those who are created in God's image, have the greatest potential for physical attractiveness. The Bible goes so far as to say our bodies are the temple of God. That makes them important indeed. But the church has typically distanced itself from making much reference to the care, maintenance, and well-being of our physical bodies, judging that the soul is somehow more important. The truth is, though, that the body and soul are equally important. We need to remind each other to get in— and stay in—good physical condition, just as we must encourage each other to be spiritually healthy. I'm not saying we need to be slaves to fashion or that we should judge each other by how we look, but we do need to call each other to physical health.

How do we do that? Surprisingly, we do it by doing what the church should do best—accepting people for how they are now. A church isn't supporting someone's health when it criticizes its people or makes judgmental statements about their physical condition.

Instead, the Golden Rule applies—treat others as you would want to be treated. With respect and dignity. If someone in your church asks for your help with a weight problem, be there to support them in their struggle (and for most people it is a struggle). Don't try to control their eating. Each person needs to be responsible for what goes into his or her own mouth. I emphasize this because one common problem of many of my overweight friends is the issue of control in their life. All of us need to be in control of our own bodies when it comes to when and what we eat.

This doesn't mean that a church can't make it easier for overweight people in their group. When there's a potluck, think about providing some low-fat dishes (raw or steamed vegetables, baked potatoes with a nonfat topping, and broiled chicken breasts). Think about fresh fruit skewers instead of pieces of pie for a celebration. Instead of ice cream sundaes maybe try fruit smoothies made from fruit and nonfat or low-fat yogurt. No one—not even the thin ones in our midst—need any extra fat or refined sugar.

And then remember that each person is different. Each one of us has his own story when it comes to weight management. Sometimes we forget that. In fact, in our culture, there is way too much prejudice against people who are heavy, and those acts and feeling of unkindness often do not stop at the door of the church. People tend not to want to get to know an overweight person because they seem to be uncomfortable in their presence. But I encourage you as you walk this exciting spiritual pathway to weight loss not to allow anyone's waistline or dress size to stop you from befriending them. Each person, regardless of his or her weight, has a special, often moving, story worth discovering and listening to.

> "The biggest disease today is not leprosy or cancer. It is the feeling of being uncared for, unwanted, of being deserted and alone."
> –Mother Teresa

KATHY'S STORY

A fault-mender is better than a fault-finder.

Kathy grew up in a traditional Christian family. Her mother taught Sunday School and her father was Sunday School superintendent. Because of this, they often sent the message to Kathy that she was supposed to be a "witness" to other children. They worried excessively about the clothes she wore, the friends she made, the way she performed in school. The message was very clear—she needed to look the part.

It was no surprise that early in childhood she found an effective way to hide her feelings. She performed this emotionally destructive high-wire assignment by learning to become a people-pleaser. If her parents wanted her to be perfect, then she would become perfect by neither thinking nor feeling. Emotionally, Kathy ceased to exist. When I asked her to talk to me about her life, it was as if the cat suddenly had her tongue. She sat there in bewildered silence. "I really can't say. I just don't know." Kathy had been married for 23 years, and from outward appearances her family seemed happy: They were involved in church, community life, and the PTA. But as she slowly began to open up, she confessed that she'd always felt disconnected from everyone—

never able to bridge the gap, never able to be close to her husband, and always finding herself distant from her children. There was a constant, terrible emptiness that kept knocking away inside, a void that started early in Kathy's childhood.

With her noncommunicative father who expected her to be the model child, Kathy was given a huge burden to bear. She never had the privilege of sharing what little courage she had with the ones who were responsible for bringing her into the world. Since this disallowed her from making friends with herself, she felt terribly alone in a darkening world. She never remembered getting a hug from her father, not even on her birthday, at Christmas, or when she was baptized at the age of ten. Now, grossly overweight at age 43, she looked back at that rejection with adult eyes, fearful of opening what she said might be a Pandora's box of pain she'd be unable to deal with. Yes, she wanted to lose weight, but, "What does my father and my background have to do with it?" she asked.

When I asked Kathy to talk to me about her current intimate relationships, she froze, unable to speak or move. She sat there as if in shock. I broke the ice and suggested that perhaps she had numbed the last four decades of pain with food, and that she may not really have any intimate friendships; that she had coped the best she could given her limited emotional resources, but that she was not a defective human being because she'd responded in this way.

As I spoke, she raised her bowed head slowly, and with tears flowing said, "Yes, that it was probably all true." She had been a lost soul for most of her life, simply hoping that it would one day get better. For Kathy, the word intimacy had too narrow a definition. She thought of it as only the physical act of sex, which never had been satisfying. It was no surprise that her sexual side was also disconnected, dutiful, frightening, devoid of desire, and light-years away from intimacy.

When I shared with Kathy that the real definition of intimacy was simply feeling close to someone, her immediate response was "I can't do that." I reminded her that she'd been doing it for years: choosing to be intimate with food rather than get close to people. She said how selfish she must be for her actions. I helped her see that she wasn't selfish at all, but that this was her way of adjusting to getting her unmet emotional needs cared for.

Kathy desperately needed to be loved and nurtured. As an adult woman, she'd tried to find that nurturing back in the church. But it never happened. She did not know how to reach out to anyone while still being the "perfect" Christian, and no one dared reach out to her.

Once the coping pattern had been established early in her life, it was relatively easy for her to continue to use food as a coping mechanism when she reached adulthood. Even in her coping, she'd been a "good girl." She hadn't gone the route of alcohol, drugs, promiscuity, and other forms of rebellion as so many of her friends had done. Food was her friend, her confidant. She did her best to keep most of her co-addictive behavior in the socially acceptable category: her endless watching of television, obsessively cleaning house, drinking diet colas—as many as six to eight cans a day—and eventually secretly hiding the empty cans because it was getting so expensive and increasingly difficult to lie about.

Kathy had become one of the most intimate persons on the planet, but it was an intimacy with safe, noncombative, nonintimate objects. She joined the occasional small-group Bible study, but she only would last two or three sessions, and she was gone. Getting close to people was too frightening. At church, she only attended large, impersonal gatherings, hoping to remain invisible. But even that was difficult. So she moved her family from the small fellowship they'd attended for years to a larger one where she felt she could hide more effectively.

If Kathy did attend any intimate social event at church or in the community, her tension would build to such intensity that she immediately would go home and begin binging on food. Food—lots of food in a short period of time—was the only thing that gave her joy. Food was her clandestine lover and her friend, her only true intimate in life.

She had discovered a miracle drug to numb her pain, and no doctor's prescription was required. It all seemed so safe. As long as she continued to mask her inner anguish with mounds of food and the layers of fat they produced, she would never find out who she was or become the person God intended her to be.

THE IMPERFECT FAMILY

God doesn't want anyone to fake perfection; it isn't our perfection that counts but the condition of our hearts.

Fortunately, when Kathy came to the realization that she needed help, her problems did not seem so insurmountable. She admitted she wasn't perfect. She gave up trying to be perfect. And then something happened. People seemed warmer to the "new Kathy." She revealed some of her imperfections, and no one criticized her. In fact, they shared some of their own struggles with her. Slowly, Kathy was able to make a few friends in her church.

In my conversations with her, we discussed that the church is a family filled with imperfect people. God doesn't want anyone to fake perfection (no one really believes it anyway). Besides, it isn't our perfection that counts but the condition of our hearts.

In my many years of counseling overweight people, I have come away with one solid conviction—the most important gift we can provide is simple, loving acceptance. Whether the relationship is friend to friend, lover to lover, or parent to child, acceptance is the single most important gift of all. That's why, in the next chapter, I am going to address the issue of raising our children with acceptance. That one ingredient alone will help our next generation understand that it truly is possible to live healthier, happier, and godlier lives.

The Undernourished Children over There Meet the Overstuffed Children over Here

*"Let no one despise your youth, but set the
believers an example in speech and conduct,
in love, in faith, in purity."*
1 Timothy 4:12

OUR CHILDREN—MIRRORS OF OURSELVES?

*The true children's rhyme should be, "Sticks
and stones may break my bones, but words
can hurt worse."*

W hat about our children? We now know that almost a quarter of all children in the United States are overweight. The unfortunate prediction is that in most cases these children will grow up to become overweight adults, who will have overweight children, who will have overweight—even obese—offspring. We find this true in church homes as well as unchurched homes. This is one classic example of the "sins" of the parents being visited on the children and even on the grandchildren.

What causes this inappropriate friendship with food? If you are a parent or grandparent who is concerned about a child's weight, I'd suggest you re-read some of the previous chapters. Many of the examples I've provided indicate how children's relationship with food can be improved by having a more solid relationship with their parents. In many cases, grandparents can make a huge contribution in helping their grandkids to feel accepted and loved.

As usual, the media needs to get their knuckles rapped a bit right here, because they need to assume their share of the blame for what has been called the "addictive" language of some of their programming and the commercials they carry. Anyone prone to a food disorder will be even further seduced by everything from the Big Mac attack, the "I can't believe I ate the whole thing" thing, and the "No one can eat just one" genre of commercials. Madison Avenue knows what it's doing, and while they make us laugh, we're dying a slow death in the process.

In my practice, I see both children and adults who've already been on several diets, and who've consumed more than their share of diet pills. They've been ridiculed for being fat and laughed at for being "abnormal." Children, in particular, have had it difficult. They've been called "whale," "big butt," "tubby," and "thunder thighs" by those who have never known the emotional pain of being the recipient of such attacks. Obesity is fast becoming an American tragedy, and until we get the message of the life-saving importance of healthy weight loss across to the community as a whole, our problem will only be exacerbated in the days ahead.

For anyone with a weight challenge—child or adult—I suggest the following five critical steps as tentative moves toward getting on—and staying on—the spiritual path to weight loss:

• **Honesty.** When you promise to deliver, deliver it. Be a person of your word. I cannot emphasize enough how important this is for adults who deal with children. Make sure your children or grandchildren know they can take you at your word.

• **Affection.** If your child has a weight problem, your boy or girl needs to be held, cuddled, and cherished. This unrushed attention is more valuable than you'll ever know. It's one way you show your child that his or her physical body is acceptable, not something to be ashamed of or ignored. A healthy relationship with our body begins in childhood.

- **Safety.** Be with people who are safe—emotionally, physically, and sexually. Shout this message loud and clear to your children. Show the child you love that they can depend on you to value their safety.

- **Boundaries.** Let others know how important boundaries are for you. It's OK to draw a line in the emotional sand. Children, especially, need to set some boundaries and have them set.

- **Structure.** One child playing on the school playground was heard complaining to her teacher, "Do we really have to do what we want to do today?" I continue to hear adults cry out for the same kind of direction. We all need structure, appropriate traditions, and a sense that some things are going to be the same day after day.

Some of you reading these words will want to turn to the child you love and make some changes in the way you relate to that child. I encourage you in this. Those changes can make a world of difference to the boy or girl in your life. Others will read these words and wonder how your own childhood problems may have contributed to your current weight problems. You may even be discovering that what you learned as a child may not have prepared you to live a happy, effective life at all. Even more on your mind might be the message that unless you are able to make critical changes with your own children, they too may be heading in an unhappy, overweight direction, carrying the terrible cycle of obesity to the next generation.

SIGNS OF CHILDHOOD TROUBLE

You cannot lift your children to a higher level than the one on which you live yourself.

◆

Although on the surface the following list of early childhood messages may seem wonderful—perhaps even saintly to you—they may actually be a series of small time bombs waiting to detonate in a child's later life. These messages might come from parents, teachers (even Sunday School teachers), pastors, grandparents—in short, any adult with influence in a child's life. If you currently love and work with children, I'd ask you to read the following list several times. These messages can become explosive devices; watch out for messages that tell children they should:

- always appear as if they have it all together.
- be brave and hide their true feelings of fear.
- always put others first and themselves last.
- not show tears when they are crying inside.

- believe that cleaning their dinner plate will save the life of a starving child overseas.
- never be seen making mistakes.

If you are pawning these ideas off on yourself or your children, please take a good look at the message you are conveying. Every example is a terrible put-down of the human spirit. As you learn to take the risk of appreciating who you are, help your child do the same. The greatest gift you can give your child is the encouragement to become the person God intended him or her to be.

PAM'S STORY

It all starts with self-awareness.

Sometimes it helps to look at someone else's struggle to see the pain in your own life or the life of someone you love. That's why I share what a woman, I'll call her Pam, told me:

> DR. JANTZ, WHEN *I get angry, I start overeating. That's just what I do. I can't help it. Being angry makes me want to clean out the fridge, and binge till the cows come home.*

Perhaps you know a child whom you believe feels this way. If you were Pam's mother or father, what would you do to help her? There are a couple ways to address this issue. One, we can try to change what makes Pam angry (which may be difficult, since the source of her anger may be outside of your control, and the person or persons involved may not be around to change). Or, two, we can help Pam gain a more current perspective of reality and help Pam change her response to the anger. Just as Pam learned to overeat when angry—because of certain destructive programming—so can she learn to substitute new, positive behaviors for her overeating patterns.

> "If you do not express your own original ideas, if you do not listen to your own being, you will have betrayed yourself."
> –Rollo May

It all starts with self-awareness. For Pam—and for anyone—not to learn to substitute positive, confident behavior for past negative emotional programming is to live a life that may be forever out of control, where she careens emotionally from wall to wall and lives with knee-jerk reactions and decisions, with little thought for how her actions affect the ones she loves.

I find that a high percentage of compulsive eaters had great difficulty in school. Many felt they completely failed academically, with their feelings of defeat starting as early as the fifth or sixth grade. (Think about how young that is!) We've documented that during those school years many seem to turn to crutches such as food in a desperate, compulsive attempt to compensate for a poor performance in the classroom. However, their peers were often so cruel in their response to those compulsive behaviors—"Hey, chubby, can't you read?"; "Tubby, wanna do my homework for me, or are you too stupid?"—that the recipient of the abuse was at a loss to respond.

Does this describe you in any way? You may have even gone beyond food for comfort; perhaps you turned to alcohol or drugs or felt you needed high-stimulus activities to keep you interested in anything. You worked hard to get the approval you needed so you could make up for your learning disabilities. It was—and may still be—a vicious cycle for you. Your life may still be a recurring nightmare of how early childhood learning disabilities, coupled with academic troubles, have set you up for a litany of compulsive behaviors; it's time to get off that train.

FOUR HALLMARKS OF SUCCESS

*God does not comfort us to make us comfortable
but to make us comforters.*

Sometimes the problems that plague the children who are dear to us are not simple. Sometimes they suffer from attention deficit–hyperactivity disorder or some other learning disability. If so, the whole-person approach to weight loss has been effective largely because this approach encourages people not to use their disability as an excuse to "fail with dignity." I will share the story of one such young woman, I'll call her Clara:

> I STILL REMEMBER *that day 12 years ago. I
> looked in the mirror, and I didn't like what I
> saw. I wanted desperately to look better. It was
> pretty embarrassing, but I could actually wear
> my boyfriend's jeans. I was Miss Chubby. I
> would even buy clothes bigger than I needed,
> because I knew I'd fill them out eventually.
> One day I said, That's it. I'm going to do this.
> I sat down and wrote out what I wanted to
> look like, how I wanted to feel, the kinds of
> clothes I wanted to wear, along with a long list*

of the kinds of personality traits I'd like to have. Being friendly, positive, and kind to others and serving people and God were just a few of my goals. I kept my list of objectives with me at all times and read it each night before I went to bed.

BUT I NEED TO BACK UP *a bit with my story.* My mother died when I was 11, and her death devastated me. I have never known such depression of heart and mind. This new sound of loneliness shattered my already fragile world as I withdrew into a shell where there was only room for Clara. The trauma of losing my mother drove me toward a long, painful, intimate friendship with food.

"HOW ARE YOU HOLDING UP, *Clara?*" People at church would ask me. "Oh, just fine. Doing great," I'd lie, torn up inside and wishing I could die. That was when I was in the sixth grade. My dad did what he could to raise me, and he gave me the best home he could. But I'd lost my mother and my friend. It did not go well with me for several years following. I longed for someone to mother me. But there was no one around—no one who looked inside my shell and saw my desperate *situation. Then, just three months before my high school graduation, my father died. I couldn't understand it. I was all alone, with no parents, no one really to understand me, and with no real friends except the food that I'd adopted as my only means of survival. With the fear, hurt, and pain of my loss, I ate and ate and ate . . . and gained and gained and gained.*

I REMEMBER WALKING *into a Christian bookstore one evening, looking for a book on how to deal with loneliness, but all the salespersons were busy, so I just wandered around, looking for something on the shelves to get me through. I found nothing, so I just left, disappearing into the cold, rainy Northwest night that only added to my sadness and fear.*

I TURNED ON THE SWITCH. *OK, Clara, let's get going here. Fortunately, I was exposed at that time to the whole-person approach, so I knew up front that my new weight-loss program would not be about dieting, rigid exercising regimens, or diet pills. Been there, done that. None of it worked. I can only describe my encounter with this new approach to weight loss as a beautiful, painful process. It wasn't* always easy. In fact, it took me a long time to learn control and discipline.

I EVEN CHANGED MY TRAFFIC *pattern for eating at school. I had always eaten in the school cafeteria where I could heap all the food I wanted on my plate three times a day—which I did, three times a day. Now, with my new weight-loss program, I decided to go to the student union cafeteria, where they would give me a pre-dished, sensible portion of food. I simply took what was offered. This taking control of my eating habits was one of the first things I learned to do. I was finally making healthy, prepared choices because I wanted to do it.*

I FOUND IT AWKWARD *when I started to lose weight, because people would say, "Hey Clara, you on a diet or something?" Well, I wasn't on a diet, but how could I say, "No, I'm losing weight because I'm dealing with the stuff in my life, like guilt, fear, and anger, blah, blah, blah." They would be long gone before I'd finished my speech. So I learned to say, "No diet. I'm just cutting back." That felt good. Just cutting back, which was true.*

I WISH I COULD TELL YOU *it was all roses from then on. It wasn't. I don't know how many* times I fell off the wagon. My greatest vice was sugar. I had been a "sugaraholic" ever since I could remember, and the urge for the sweet stuff never left me. I'd start with one piece of candy, and before long the whole box would be history. It was only when I remembered my long-term goals of how I wanted to look, feel, and be that I would drift back on course.

LITTLE BY LITTLE, *I learned more about who I really was. Unconnected. Addicted to jewelry, nice clothes, cars, and other gadgets that shine and glitter. For so long I didn't know what I needed to bring into my life to make me whole. If we who are overweight appear lost, it's because we are lost. Our behaviors are illogical and unpredictable. The world of disordered eating is a darkened universe that others do not understand. It's a world not based on logic or reason. If logic were the key, we'd all just go on diets, be thin, and be loved by everyone. The truth is that without coming to grips with our past, we will never stop abusing food. We just can't do it.*

HERE'S WHY: GUILT *has no calories. Anger has no fat. Fear has no cholesterol. It's when we stuff these unresolved emotions into the already cluttered basements of our minds that they become time bombs waiting to detonate who knows when. This was true for me. They were truly time bombs with short fuses, and they went off with painful regularity.*

WELL, I'VE GONE ON TOO LONG. *But I want to close by saying this. I am at peace with myself today—with my body, my appearance, my personality, my relationships, and my work. I have developed the confidence to know that it's OK to communicate my needs. I have wonderful people in my life who respond to me and my needs in ways that help me feel safe. Safety, for me, is still a big word.*

BUT MOST OF ALL *I'm at peace. I still have my share of conflicts and struggles, but my life now is all about peace and contentment. I have lost my obsession for food because I have dealt with the real obsessions in my life. It's been 12 years since I lost those 40 pounds. I never expect to see them again.*

I've shared Clara's story with you because it shows what a difference a caring adult can make in the life of a

> A listening ear is the most precious gift you can give a child.

child. The gift we give to a child when we give them our caring support is an invaluable gift. Your love and acceptance can make sure that a child will never even need to head down that path to weight loss because a loved child is a child who knows peace and self-acceptance.

Close Your Eyes and Make a Wish

*"And the one who was seated on the throne said,
'See, I am making all things new.'"*
Revelation 21:5

HEAVEN ON EARTH

*The journey of a thousand miles begins with
a single step.*

I can hear your question now: "Do I have to wait for heaven to be the thin person I want to be?" If you learn nothing else from this book, I want you to learn this one thing: The answer to that question is no. You can start becoming the wonderful person you already are right now. This is not a reduced-fat pie-in-the-sky kind of dream. This is here and now in your life. The spiritual path to weight loss is a road that leads you deeper into an understanding of the special person God has created you to be. That path will engage your talents, help you take control and responsibility for your own life, and put to rest some of the troubles of your past.

And that path is right in front of you. You don't need to buy expensive equipment, costly and exclusive diet foods, pills, or any thing else. You already have everything you need to stay the spiritual course to weight loss. Just pick up your feet and keep on walking, just as you've done since chapter one.

I'm not saying that the path will always be smooth. It won't. There will be gnarled roots of old problems that will rise up on that path, causing you to stumble. People, perhaps even your best friends, will try to show you an easier way—a path that demands little or no commitment to weight loss and one that does not involve the whole person. When confronted with these distractions, remember your commitment and continue on. There may also be crevices for you in the path where you will need to build a bridge so that you can walk to the other side. Build that bridge. Do what it takes to get across the chasm. There may be cliffs on one side and mountains on the other. Don't be distracted. Just keep walking, and keep on listening to your heavenly Father who wants you to stay on your spiritual path—the road less traveled.

To help you continue to put one foot in front of the other, I want to tell you something a wise person once told me. Actually, it's a story—one that will help keep your mind focused on one step at a time, and not the many challenges that surely lie ahead:

How Much Do You Want It?

If you aren't honest with yourself, how can you be honest with others?

❧

A brilliant woman pianist once gave an intimate performance for a small group of society women in the sun-drenched library of a large country estate. Later, while dessert was being served, a guest approached the pianist, gushing, "I would give anything in the world to play as you play." The virtuoso looked at the woman for a moment and said, "I'm sorry, madam, but I don't think you would." You could have heard a paper napkin drop on the plush carpet beneath their feet. Red-faced, but not one to be daunted, the guest tried again, quietly this time, "But really, I truly would give anything to play the piano with the skill that you do."

The pianist, realizing she had not successfully made her point, said, "No, my dear, I'm afraid you really wouldn't. If you would, you might play better than I, at least equally as well. Yes, you'd give anything except your time, the one thing it takes to be good. You would not sit on a bench practicing hour after hour, day after day while your friends were out having fun, enjoying parties such as this, and otherwise getting on with their lives."

Then she smiled, "Please don't get me wrong. I hope you understand that I'm not criticizing you. I don't even know you. I'm just telling you when you say you'd give anything to play the piano as I do, that in your heart of hearts you don't really mean it. You really don't mean it at all."

When I heard that story I said, Wow, that's one honest woman. The talented pianist knew that in music only a few percent succeed at what they attempt, even though most will say they want to be great, famous, and well-paid. But in reality, only the dedicated few will realize their cherished ambitions. Why? Because to be an accomplished musician requires time, patience, preparation, hard work, focus, and the ability to postpone pleasures that do not lead to desired goals.

Does all this sound familiar? Of course it does because we, too, have tried our best to be honest enough in this book to say that among those who lose weight, only a few succeed. Does that mean you should not try? That you should throw your hands up in despair, crying, "I'll never be able to do it!"? That you should go back to the insanity of diets and infomercial hype and model the 98 percent who will never make it? Only you can answer those questions. But my sincere hope is that you are now convinced that you do have the determination, dedication, desire, and direction to make the changes necessary to put you on the path to weight loss once and for all, for the rest of your life.

> "You gain strength, courage and confidence by every experience in which you really stop to look fear in the face. You must do the thing you cannot do."
>
> –Eleanor Roosevelt

WHAT ARE YOU BUILDING?

Without knowing the true goal, you'll never be able to get there.

As you come to the close of this book—and I thank you from the bottom of my heart for spending time with me as we've traveled this path together—it's my hope that you have edged ever closer to understanding the depths of your own personal sense of freedom. Think, for a moment, about your old patterns. In the past you may have been glued to a late-night infomercial touting the latest fad diet program, or you saw a Hollywood star demonstrating a piece of expensive, all-purpose exercise equipment that was supposed to be the *pièce de résistance*, and you felt you just had to have it or die. However, if you purchased it, was it all you'd hoped it would be? You may have said you wanted tight buns, greater stamina, a rippling "six pack" of abs, bulging biceps, and a champion's chest—all good in themselves. Did you really get all you wanted? Did the products make you a happier, more fulfilled person even if you did reach some of your goals? Has the weight-loss game ended yet?

In your heart of hearts ask yourself, What do I really want in my life? Do I want a body to rival the latest cover girl on my favorite magazine, or do I want happiness and a deep sense of inner joy? Do I really want "buns of steel," or would I be happier with lasting peace of mind and good friends and the firmer buns and trimmer tummy as simple byproducts of my exercise regimen? You already know that unfulfilled expectations invariably lead to guilt, which leads to depression, which leads to compulsive behavior, which leads to using food for comfort—comfort to get out of the depression, which leads back to anger at ourselves that we did it again! This anger paralyzes us with fear that we're never going to be able to do this...and the beat goes on.

A friend once told me this story:

A woman approached two stonemasons working on a rather large project. She paused to ask each man, "What are you doing?" The first man looked at the woman, and said hurriedly, "Lady, can't you see? I'm laying bricks!" She turned to the other workman, and asked, "And what, may I ask, are you doing?" He paused for a moment and, with a faraway look in his eye, said, "Madam, I'm building a beautiful cathedral which will shoot its spires high into the heavens, bringing glory to God for generations to come."

Before you step out on the spiritual path to weight loss, ask yourself: What am I doing? Laying bricks? Going through the motions of life, reliving past hurts, blaming others, and taking periodic guilt trips? Or are you building a landmark of beauty by becoming the person God created you to be? It is my prayer that the pages of this book have given you the blueprints to create such a building. If that is what I've placed into your hands with these pages, then you have given me the greatest gift an author could ever hope for. I wish you the best today, tomorrow, and forever as you enthusiastically start down the spiritual path of weight loss.

STEPS ALONG THE WAY

*"For life is more than food, and the body
more than clothing...."*
Luke 12:23

Since the way won't always be smooth, I want to give you a few suggestions on how to dig out some of those gnarled old roots that may try to block your path:

First, don't listen to the media messages you hear about what is beautiful and what is not. You'll become frustrated and discouraged. In fact, I sometimes recommend to people that they do more than close their ears. Here's what I told a friend who was trying to lose weight:

Go through some current or past issues of *Vogue, Cosmopolitan, Redbook, Muscle and Fitness,* and other "beautiful body" magazines and tear out every page that reinforces a negative role about your body—one that suggests you need to need to be rail-thin, pumped, or well-endowed in the right places to feel good about yourself. Place these pages in a stack and tie them up. Then take them outside where it's safe—to the seashore, or to a barbecue pit—and burn them. Watch the false messages go up in smoke, along with the negative programming that up until now created your self-sabotaging behavior. Then, whenever you feel you are being lured into the "glamour" trap, remember that the symbols of that deceit have already been consumed and are no longer a threat to you because you are now walking the spiritual path to weight loss.

As you engage in your daily commitment to lose weight by becoming an emotionally healthier, more complete person, you will need to develop a deeper love and appreciation for yourself—the person God created so uniquely. With that in mind complete the following:

For me to truly love and appreciate who I am, I need:

For me to believe in my heart that I am worthy of being loved, whether I'm thin or not, I must:

For me to become more open and loving, I need to:

YOUR NEW LIFE

Life's best outlook is a prayerful outlook. Prayer will keep you on the spiritual path to weight loss.

People who lose weight and keep it off learn the importance of removing toxins from their lives—toxins that have subverted their growth and kept them from becoming the caring men and women God created them to be.

As these terrible toxins are flushed from their system, they begin to learn the importance of intimacy. Their relationship with their spouse deepens and becomes more meaningful. They find themselves at home in social situations where they were never comfortable before. They learn to risk. They learn to forgive, and they spend more time building bridges of friendship than they do destroying them.

Is this what overweight people wanted when they began their holistic approach to losing weight? No, it wasn't. Virtually every person who comes to The Center for weight counseling simply wants to lose weight. What each one soon discovers, however, is that he or she is wonderfully and beautifully made—so intricate, in fact, that the challenge of weight loss becomes a mere byproduct of becoming a growing, giving, loving person—one who understands and chooses to be close to others, no longer afraid. This is what true intimacy is all about.

If you are ready to take the steps I've suggested in this book toward your adventure of a lifetime, you must remain open to the moment. Promise yourself you will never fail to keep discovering the person you were designed to be. The good news is that joy unspeakable is ready to come your way when you open your heart to see, touch, and feel the goodness of others, to experience your own depth, and to make it your business today—and every day—to nourish your spirit, even as you shower those around you with love and compassion. People who journey down the spiritual path to weight loss know what it means to draw closer to others: the willingness to let others see the real you—the big, generous, loving heart you hold inside.

If you take that secret with you, you are taking the steps along your special spiritual path of weight loss. You recognize the importance of being authentically you, the you God created you to be. You will no longer let your fears stop you or trip you up. You now have the confidence to take one step, and then another, and then another. That's what paths are for—to be taken one footstep at a time.

As you've read this book, I hope you've come to understand the love God has for you. It is this love that will give you the courage to step forth. Reach out to others. Ask for support. Learn to reveal yourself to those close to you. I know it takes courage to begin and even more courage to continue the pilgrimage. I'm proud of you for taking these first steps. God bless you, and keep you. May the winds be always at your back as you take your own unique spiritual path to weight loss—a spiritual exercise that brings glory to God.